CANCER ETIOLOGY, DIAGNOSIS AND TREATMENTS

HODGKIN'S AND T-CELL LYMPHOMA

DIAGNOSIS, TREATMENT OPTIONS AND PROGNOSIS

CANCER ETIOLOGY, DIAGNOSIS AND TREATMENTS

Additional books in this series can be found on Nova's website under the Series tab.

Additional e-books in this series can be found on Nova's website under the e-book tab.

CANCER ETIOLOGY, DIAGNOSIS AND TREATMENTS

HODGKIN'S AND T-CELL LYMPHOMA

DIAGNOSIS, TREATMENT OPTIONS AND PROGNOSIS

WARREN K. HARVEY
AND
RANDALL M. JACOBS
EDITORS

New York

Library of Congress Cataloging-in-Publication Data

ISBN 978-1-62257-478-0
Library of Congress Control Number: 2012942451

Published by Nova Science Publishers, Inc. † New York

CONTENTS

PREFACE

In this book, the authors present current research in the study of the diagnosis, treatments options and prognosis of both Hodgkin's and T-Cell lymphomas, gathered from across the globe. Topics discussed include the pathology and pathogenesis of Hodgkin's lymphoma; total skin electron beam therapy in the treatment of cutaneous T-Cell lymphoma; HIV-associated T-Cell lymphoma; critical mass hypothesis of T-Cell responses and its application in the treatment of T-Cell lymphoma; combined modality therapy, the short term benefits and long term toxicities in Hodgkin's lymphoma; and enteropathy-associated T-Cell lymphoma diagnosis and risk-stratification.

Chapter 1 - The histopathological and fine-needle aspiration (FNA) cytologic diagnosis of Hodgkin's lymphoma (HL) is based on demonstration of the so called pathognomonic mononucleated Hodgkin's and bi- to multinucleated Reed-Sternberg (HRS) cells among reactive cellular component composed of lymphocytes, benign histiocytes, neutrophils and eosinophils. Hodgkin's lymphoma (HL) is one of the most common lymphomas in the developed world with an incidence of approximately three per 100,000 person-years but it is uncommon in the Far-East countries as compared to rest of the world and relatively uncommon in Sub-Saharan African countries. When the reported frequency in the Far-East countries was compared with the rest of the world, it exceeded 20% in none of the reports from the Far East countries, as opposed to 15 (68.2%) from rest of the world (p=0.00002). When Sub-Saharan African countries were compared with rest of the non-Far-East countries of the world, it was observed that the frequency of HL exceeded 20% in 2 (28.6%) of the Sub-Saharan African countries and in13 (86.7%) of the 15 other counties (p=0.01355). Nearly five decades ago Hodgkin's lymphoma, then known as Hodgkin's disease (HD) was categorized under Rye classification into lymphocytic predominant (LP), nodular sclerosis (NS), mixed cellularity (MC) and lymphocytic depletion (LD) sub-types. Analysis of 33 reports on Rye classification from various countries revealed that the median percentages for LP, NS, MC and LD subtypes were 10.0%, 58.5%, 26.0% and 2.6%, respectively, from the developed economies and the corresponding figures from the developing countries were 9.5%, 29.4%, 44.1% and 8.9%, respectively. In NS subtype, the frequency exceeded 50% in significantly higher number of reports from the developed (9 of 13, 69.2%) than developing countries (3 of 20, 15.0%, p= 0.00281). A reverse trend was observed in MC subtype wherein frequency exceeding 30% of cases were compared (23.1% of the reports in developed vs. 90.0% in the developing world, p=0.00016). However, there was no significant difference between the developed and developing countries in respect of LP and LD subtypes when the number of reports with frequency exceeding 10% were compared (p=1.0000, and =0.70059, respectively).

The sub-classification of HL into LP, MC, and LD in histology as well as cytology depends on relative proportion of neoplastic HRS cells and reactive cellular components. In nodular sclerosis type of HL, islands of neoplastic cells including a special type of R-S cells called lacunar cells and reactive cell components are surrounded by collagenous bands, which are not appreciated in cytologic preparations leading to limitation of cytology in the diagnosis of NS subtype. HL is an unusual malignancy in which the malignant cells are much less (about 1% cells in tumor tissue) compared to reactive cell components. In the past, various possibilities put forth regarding nature of Hodgkin's disease were inflammatory, neoplastic, autoimmune reaction and an intermediate stage between inflammatory & neoplastic lesions. HRS cells were traditionally believed to be abnormal reticulum cells. With the advent of immunological markers in 1970s, three candidates emerged as possible sources of HRS cells: T-lymphocytes, B-lymphocytes and macrophages; interdigitating reticulm cells and early progenitor myeloid cells subsequently joined the membership club of progenitor cells. Based on observation of R-S cell and T-lymphocyte interaction, and stepwise cytolysis of R-S cells in scanning electron microscopic study, it was proposed that Hodgkin's disease was a war between T-lymphocytes and transformed macrophages; the various histological subtypes depended upon the outcome of this war. During this period, the understanding of nature of cells in the formation of non-Hodgkin's lymphoma (NHL) led to the emergence of a number of classifications and wide range of controversies was associated with it. Unlike non-Hodgkin's lymphoma, the fortress of Hodgkin's lymphoma seemed invincible in seventies through eighties into early nineties. But gradually notes of dissent started to appear. In earlier reports, Reed-Sternberg-like cells were reported not only in benign lymphoproliferative conditions like reactive lymphoid hyperplasia and infectious mononucleosis, but some of nonHodgkin lymphoma subtypes, e.g., chronic lymphocytic leukemia, mycosis fungoides, Burkitt's lymphoma, lymphoepithelioid lymphoma and immunoblastic lymphoma, and non-lymphoid malignancies like metastatic carcinoma, melanoma, sarcomas and germ cell tumors revealed presence of RS-like cells. It was subsequently found that some subtypes of non-Hodgkin lymphoma like anaplastic large cell lymphoma (ALCL), T-cell-histiocytic-rich B-cell lymphoma (TCHRBCL), and pleomorphic peripheral T-cell lymphoma were most commonly misdiagnosed as Hodgkin's disease. The immunocytochemical markers like CD15, CD30, CD45, CD3 and CD20 were of help in differentiating these entities. The immunocytochemical markers for HL were CD15+, CD30+, CD45-, B-, T-, and EMA-. ALCL were CD15-, CD30+, CD45+, B±, T±, EMA± and Alk1 ±; later B+ cases were excluded from ALCL pool. The neoplastic cells in TCHRBCL were CD15-, CD30-, CD45+, CD3-, CD20+, EMA-; the accompanying rich lymphoid cell population was CD3+ and histiocytes were CD68+. With the separation of these entities, the empire of Hodgkin's disease started disintegrating. New immunohistochemical and molecular studies proved that the neoplastic cells in Hodgkin's disease was of B-cell origin and it was renamed as Hodgkin's lymphoma. In the WHO classification of Tumors of Hematopoietic and Lymphoid Tissue, Hodgkin's lymphoma was classified as nodular lymphocytic predominant HL and classical HL which was in turn classified into lymphocyte-rich, mixed cellular, lymphocytic depleted and nodular sclerosis subtypes. At present there is compelling evidence that HRS cells are clonal B-cells that have lost their B-cell phenotype. Whereas, classical HL is associated with crippling mutation of immunoglobulin genes, which prevents the production of a functional immunoglobulin molecule, the nodular lymphocytic predominance HL is associated with ongoing immunoglobulin gene hypermutation but absence of crippling mutation in their immunoglobulin genes. Mature B-cells lacking B-cell receptors would normally die by apoptosis. The rescue of Hodgkin cells and R-S cells from apoptosis is a key event in HL pathogenesis. Hodgkin cells and R-S cells express a number of receptors (at least six receptors that belong to TNF receptor family) that regulate tumor cell survival. Epstein-Barr virus (EBV), which was initially implicated in the pathogenesis of Burkitt's lymphoma, was found to be associated with other nonlymphoid malignancies (e.g., nasoparyngeal carcinoma and gastric carcinoma) and lymphoid neoplasms (B- and T-cell NHL). HL in varying proportions (ranged 26.1%to 93.8%, with a median 46.8%) was found to be associated with EBV in different studies. The escape from apoptosis and transcriptional reprogramming of HRS cells are interlinked and appear central to pathogenesis of HL. It is likely that EBV plays a role in reprogramming and survival through dysregulation of several signaling networks and transcription factors. As regards the reactive cellular infiltrate in HL, there is increased number of T-cells (CD4 and NKT subsets), decreased B-cells, and increased regulatory T-cells in comparision with reactive hyperplasia of lymph node; the tumor associated macrophages in HL are of prognostic importance. As it stands today, most of the cases of NHL and HL cases can be diagnosed based on cyto/histomorphology, immunocytochemistry, cytogenetic and molecular studies. However, there were some grey zone lymphomas, which do not exactly fall into either HL or NHL sub-types like ALCL and TCHRBCL. It appears that Hodgkin lymphoma and its pathogenesis is still in a stage of evolution and only future will tell when this turbulent phase will settle down.

Chapter 2 - Cutaneous T-cell Lymphoma is a relatively rare dermatological disease, with whole body symptomatology. The organ being mostly affected is the skin, without excluding internal organ involvement in progressed stages of the disease. For the cure of this type of lymphoma, several treatments have been employed. Fractionated irradiation of the whole skin surface, by high energy electrons, is one of the suggested therapeutic courses, either as exclusive or supplementary treatment. This method of external radiation therapy is commonly referred to in bibliography as Total Skin Electron Beam (TSEB) treatment, Every currently applied TSEB technique is based on a fundamental principle: the utilization of a homogeneous broad electron beam that can cover the patient in height and width. Due to their physical properties, high energy electrons (4-9 MeV) are appropriate for treating superficial lesions, while sufficiently wide fields can be generated by increasing the distance of the patient from the electron source (SSD > 3m). Such a beam can be produced by every commercially available linear accelerator, equipped with electron scattering foils. Nevertheless, the establishment of a total skin treatment protocol in a radiation therapy unit is a rather complex procedure. Unconventional patient positioning increases the number and frequency of quality checks. In addition, specially designed equipment is necessary for patient immobilization and support. Subsequently, only a limited number of health centers worldwide provide this kind of radiation therapy. Existing TSEB techniques are categorized depending on the manner of irradiation (standing, rotating-on-platform or reclined patient) and the number of required fields for total skin coverage. Despite the variety of irradiation setups, over 80% of the clinics already providing TSEB have adopted a "six dual-field" arrangement. A critical safety aspect of TSEB is to minimize exposure of the patient to contaminating Bremsstrahlung radiation, derived from electrons interacting with parts of the linear accelerator's head. Therapeutic doses range between 20-40 cGy on skin, with the majority of centers prescribing an average of 36 cGy in a 9 week treatment scheme. In the authors'institute, a "six dual-field" TSEB technique was developed, following international guidelines of radiation safety and dose prescription. A uniquely designed immobilization system was constructed by the authors'clinic, equipped with a PMMA scatterer of proper dimensions. From the first clinical trial until now, all T-cell lymphoma patients being submitted into theirtreatment protocol, presented positive preliminary results, even up to full remission of the disease in certain cases. During the six decades of its existence, Total Skin Electron Beam irradiation has proven to be a reliable and effective treatment, for cure or palliation of cutaneous T-cell lymphoma, especially in early stages of the disease.

Chapter 3 - Hodgkin lymphoma (HL) is one of the most common malignancies in adolescents and older adults, accounting for more than 10% of the cancers annually in the developed world. It has a bimodal age distribution curve with the pattern of age incidence differing by geographic location. There are epidemiological risk factors that are associated with developing HL and they include family history of lymphoma, exposure to Epstein Barr virus, socioeconomic status, residence and social contacts. Hodgkin Lymphoma can be divided into two pathologic classes which include classical HL and nodular lymphocyte predominant HL. Clinically, most patients present with painless adenopathy and a constellation of systemic symptoms such as fever, weight loss, or night sweats that are considered B symptoms and are important for treatment and prognosis. Diagnosis of HL relies on a physical examination and history, computed topography scans along with newer nuclear medicine imaging fluorodeoxyglucose positron emission tomography (FDG-PET). Standard treatment includes risk adapted chemotherapy and radiotherapy. Treatment for recurrent or resistant disease includes conventional chemo and radiotherapy and hematopoietic stem cell transplant. Through prognosis remains very favorable with over 70% of patients being cured of their disease there are a number of adverse long term effects from therapy. Potential adverse long term toxicities can include cardiopulmonary dysfunction, gonadal dysfunction, infertility, thyroid disease and secondary malignancies. Modern era treatment aims to decrease toxicity from therapy while advancing the cure rate.

Chapter 4 - Hodgkin's lymphoma (HL) is a rare monoclonal lymphoid malignancy of B-cell origin, which represents circa 12-18 % of all lymphomas.

It shows characteristic clinical and morphological features. The disease remains localised for a long period of time. The histological characteristics are the bilobated Hodgkin and Reed-Sternberg (HRS) cells for classical HL, and their variants the lymphocytic and hystiocytic (LandH) cells, for nodular lymphocyte predominant HL, surrounded by large, non-malignant, reactive tissue. Both pathognomonic HRS and LandH cells go through somatic hypermutation. Phenotypically HRS cells are CD15 and CD30 positive, while LandH cells are CD20 positive. The exact etiology is still unknown, however the role of genetical, immunological and viral infection (Ebstein-Barr virus) seem important. Environmental factors might explain, why deficient response against HRS cells occurs. More than half of the HL patients have no complaints, lymphadenomegaly and hepato-splenomegaly can be seen at the time of the diagnosis, while B symptoms (fever, night sweats and loss of weight) are more specific for advanced stage. Patients suspect to HL go through a specific check-up, lymph node and bone marrow biopsy for histological diagnosis and various imaging techniques (ultrasound, X-ray, CT or, ^{18}FDG PET/CT scan) for staging. Nowadays the standard combined chemo-radiotherapy consisting of adriamycin bleomycin vinblastine dacarbazine (ABVD) regimen is expected to cure 80-85% of patients. Risk-adapted strategy involving conventional prognostic factors, such as the European Organization for Research and Treatment of Cancer (EORTC), in early and International Prognostic Score (IPS) in advanced stage HL are known to avoid over- and under-treating patients. The early identification of refractory patients by interim PET/CT may be beneficial thus further improves patient outcome and help to avoid late side effects. Combining standard care with novel epigenetic and targeted therapies (anti-CD20 and anti-CD30 antibodies) may be promising and clinical trials currently take place to assess the efficacy of these novel treatment regimes.

Chapter 5 - *T*-*c*ell *l*ymphoma (TCL) occurrence in the setting of the *a*cquired *i*mmune *d*eficiency *s*yndrome (AIDS) and human immunodeficiency virus (HIV) infection is infrequent. The vast majority of *A*IDS-*r*elated *l*ymphomas (ARL) are of B-cell origin with TCL accounting for only 1.5-3% of all cases. Epidemiologic studies, however, suggest that people living with HIV/AIDS have a 15-fold higher risk of TCL compared to comparably matched but HIV-negative cohorts. While a direct causal role for HIV in T-cell lymphomagenesis is not established, co-infection with other oncogenic viruses including Epstein-Barr virus, hepatitis-C virus, and human T-lymphotropic virus type-I have been implicated in AIDS-related TCL (ARTCL). The diversity of viral co-infections linked to the various ARTCLs is illustrative of the histopathologic and clinical heterogeneity of these various non-Hodgkin's lymphomas. Although aggressive TCL portends a poor prognosis, several novel therapies have recently been shown to have significant activity in TCL. Whether these agents can be safely used in patients with ARTCL and with similar efficacy is a question of immediate clinical relevance.

Chapter 6 - Adaptive immune responses against intracellular pathogens and cancer must find a balance between the effective elimination of target cells on one hand, and collateral damage to healthy tissues on the other. Precise and subtle timing of effector activity is vital to achieving this balance. Ligand-induced TCR down-modulation, whereby T cell receptors (TCR) are removed from the surface shortly after engagement with peptide-MHC (p-MHC), has been extensively studied over the past 20 years; however this critical process is still poorly understood, and both the underlying mechanism and its physiological significance remain unclear. Most experimental evidence supports that TCR down-modulation attenuates T cell activation by removing TCRs from the T cell surface, thereby limiting TCR signal transduction and preventing cell hyper-activation and hazardous inflammation. Here, the authors put forward a complementary hypothesis. TCRs are down-modulated after antigen presentation and remain so during the exponential phase of effector T cell expansion. Then, TCRs are re-expressed as T cell numbers reach their peak. In this way the initiation of cytotoxic responses can be synchronised with the time at which a "critical mass" of effector T cells has accumulated. Therefore, TCR down-modulation co-ordinates cytotoxic function with effector capacity, reducing the likelihood of untimely cytotoxic activity which could give rise to autoimmune disease. The authors discuss the therapeutic implications of targeting TCR down-modulation and modifying the kinetics of T cell responses, with an emphasis on their application for immunotherapy of T cell lymphoma.

Chapter 7 - Advances in the treatment of Hodgkin lymphoma (HL) led to improvement in survival outcomes. This success however, brought new challenges in dealing with long-term morbidity. The combined chemotherapy and radiation therapy (CMT) undoubtedly changed the cure rate in this once incurable disease. This approach is associated with long-term toxicities including secondary malignancies and early cardiovascular disease. This led to the launch of many trials investigating the minimal effective therapy that would reduce late toxicities without jeopardizing overall survival. Although an optimal risk stratification system is still elusive, factors such as molecular markers and interim imaging are emerging as prognostic indicators. Radiation therapy plays an important role in a subset of patients with HL, the challenge remains to identify and risk stratify therapy.

Chapter 8 - Enteropathy–Associated T-Cell Lymphoma (EATL) is an extranodal peripheral T-cell lymphoma derived from intraepithelial lymphocytes (IELs) of the intestinal mucosa that commonly involves the small intestine and is classically associated with celiac sprue. EATLs, classified by the World Health Organization (WHO) into two subtypes with distinct clinical and pathologic features, are aggressive lymphomas with a dismal prognosis. Disease- and treatment-related complications, along with chemorefractory disease, are common. Therefore, the median overall survival is less than one year, with few long-term survivors. Improved understanding of the molecular pathogenesis of EATL is greatly needed if novel therapeutic approaches are to be developed for this aggressive and poorly understood T-cell lymphoma. In this chapter the authors will review the natural history, diagnosis, risk-stratification, and treatment strategies for EATL.

In: Hodgkin's and T-Cell Lymphoma
Editors: Warren K. Harvey and Randall M. Jacobs

ISBN 978-1-62257-478-0

Chapter 1

PATHOLOGY AND PATHOGENESIS OF HODGKIN'S LYMPHOMA: ANALYSIS OF ITS STATUS OVER A PERIOD OF FIVE DECADES

Dilip K. Das*
Department of Pathology, Faculty of Medicine,
Kuwait University, Kuwait

ABSTRACT

The histopathological and fine-needle aspiration (FNA) cytologic diagnosis of Hodgkin's lymphoma (HL) is based on demonstration of the so called pathognomonic mononucleated Hodgkin's and bi- to multinucleated Reed-Sternberg (HRS) cells among reactive cellular component composed of lymphocytes, benign histiocytes, neutrophils and eosinophils. Hodgkin's lymphoma (HL) is one of the most common lymphomas in the developed world with an incidence of approximately three per 100,000 person-years but it is uncommon in the Far-East countries as compared to rest of the world and relatively uncommon in Sub-Saharan African countries. When the reported frequency in the Far-East countries was compared with the rest of the world, it exceeded 20% in none of the reports from the Far-East countries, as opposed to 15 (68.2%) from rest of the world (p=0.00002). When Sub-Saharan African countries were compared with rest of the non-Far-East countries of the world, it was observed that the frequency of HL exceeded 20% in 2 (28.6%) of the Sub-Saharan African countries and in13 (86.7%) of the 15 other counties (p=0.01355). Nearly five decades ago Hodgkin's lymphoma, then known as Hodgkin's disease (HD) was categorized under Rye classification into lymphocytic predominant (LP), nodular sclerosis (NS), mixed cellularity (MC) and lymphocytic depletion (LD) sub-types. Analysis of 33 reports on Rye classification from various countries revealed that the median percentages for LP, NS, MC and LD subtypes were 10.0%, 58.5%, 26.0% and 2.6%, respectively, from the developed economies and the corresponding figures from the developing countries were 9.5%, 29.4%, 44.1% and 8.9%,

* Address for Correspondence: Dr. Dilip K. Das, MBBS, MD, PhD, DSc, FRCPath. Department of Pathology, Faculty of Medicine, Kuwait University, P.O. Box: 24923, Safat 13110. Kuwait. Tel: 00965-25319476, Fax: 00965-25338905, E-mail: dilip76@hotmail.com.

respectively. In NS subtype, the frequency exceeded 50% in significantly higher number of reports from the developed (9 of 13, 69.2%) than developing countries (3 of 20, 15.0%, p= 0.00281). A reverse trend was observed in MC subtype wherein frequency exceeding 30% of cases were compared (23.1% of the reports in developed vs. 90.0% in the developing world, p=0.00016). However, there was no significant difference between the developed and developing countries in respect of LP and LD subtypes when the number of reports with frequency exceeding 10% were compared (p=1.0000, and =0.70059, respectively).

The sub-classification of HL into LP, MC, and LD in histology as well as cytology depends on relative proportion of neoplastic HRS cells and reactive cellular components. In nodular sclerosis type of HL, islands of neoplastic cells including a special type of R-S cells called lacunar cells and reactive cell components are surrounded by collagenous bands, which are not appreciated in cytologic preparations leading to limitation of cytology in the diagnosis of NS subtype. HL is an unusual malignancy in which the malignant cells are much less (about 1% cells in tumor tissue) compared to reactive cell components. In the past, various possibilities put forth regarding nature of Hodgkin's disease were inflammatory, neoplastic, autoimmune reaction and an intermediate stage between inflammatory & neoplastic lesions. HRS cells were traditionally believed to be abnormal reticulum cells. With the advent of immunological markers in 1970s, three candidates emerged as possible sources of HRS cells: T-lymphocytes, B-lymphocytes and macrophages; interdigitating reticulm cells and early progenitor myeloid cells subsequently joined the membership club of progenitor cells. Based on observation of R-S cell and T-lymphocyte interaction, and stepwise cytolysis of R-S cells in scanning electron microscopic study, it was proposed that Hodgkin's disease was a war between T-lymphocytes and transformed macrophages; the various histological subtypes depended upon the outcome of this war. During this period, the understanding of nature of cells in the formation of non-Hodgkin's lymphoma (NHL) led to the emergence of a number of classifications and wide range of controversies was associated with it. Unlike non-Hodgkin's lymphoma, the fortress of Hodgkin's lymphoma seemed invincible in seventies through eighties into early nineties. But gradually notes of dissent started to appear. In earlier reports, Reed-Sternberg-like cells were reported not only in benign lymphoproliferative conditions like reactive lymphoid hyperplasia and infectious mononucleosis, but some of nonHodgkin lymphoma subtypes, e.g., chronic lymphocytic leukemia, mycosis fungoides, Burkitt's lymphoma, lymphoepithelioid lymphoma and immunoblastic lymphoma, and non-lymphoid malignancies like metastatic carcinoma, melanoma, sarcomas and germ cell tumors revealed presence of RS-like cells. It was subsequently found that some subtypes of non-Hodgkin lymphoma like anaplastic large cell lymphoma (ALCL), T-cell-histiocytic-rich B-cell lymphoma (TCHRBCL), and pleomorphic peripheral T-cell lymphoma were most commonly misdiagnosed as Hodgkin's disease. The immunocytochemical markers like CD15, CD30, CD45, CD3 and CD20 were of help in differentiating these entities. The immunocytochemical markers for HL were CD15+, CD30+, CD45-, B-, T-, and EMA-. ALCL were CD15-, CD30+, CD45+, B±, T±, EMA± and Alk1 ±; later B+ cases were excluded from ALCL pool. The neoplastic cells in TCHRBCL were CD15-, CD30-, CD45+, CD3-, CD20+, EMA-; the accompanying rich lymphoid cell population was CD3+ and histiocytes were CD68+. With the separation of these entities, the empire of Hodgkin's disease started disintegrating. New immunohistochemical and molecular studies proved that the neoplastic cell in Hodgkin's disease was of B-cell origin and it was renamed as Hodgkin's lymphoma. In the WHO classification of Tumors of Hematopoietic and Lymphoid Tissue, Hodgkin's lymphoma was classified as nodular lymphocytic predominant HL and classical HL which was in turn classified into lymphocyte-rich, mixed cellular, lymphocytic depleted and nodular sclerosis subtypes. At present there is compelling evidence that HRS cells are clonal B-cells that have lost their B-cell phenotype. Whereas, classical HL is associated with crippling mutation of immunoglobulin genes, which prevents the production of a functional immunoglobulin molecule, the nodular lymphocytic predominance HL is associated with ongoing immunoglobulin gene hypermutation but absence of crippling mutation in their immunoglobulin genes. Mature B-cells lacking B-cell receptors would normally die by apoptosis. The rescue of Hodgkin cells and R-S cells from apoptosis is a key event in HL pathogenesis. Hodgkin cells and R-S cells express a number of receptors (at least six receptors that belong to TNF receptor family) that regulate tumor cell survival. Epstein-Barr virus (EBV), which was initially implicated in the pathogenesis of Burkitt's lymphoma, was found to be associated with other nonlymphoid malignancies (e.g., nasoparyngeal carcinoma and gastric carcinoma) and lymphoid neoplasms (B- and T-cell NHL). HL in varying proportions (ranged 26.1%to 93.8%, with a median 46.8%) was found to be associated with EBV in different studies. The escape from apoptosis and transcriptional reprogramming of HRS cells are interlinked and appear central to pathogenesis of HL. It is likely that EBV plays a role in reprogramming and survival through dysregulation of several signaling networks and transcription factors. As regards the reactive cellular infiltrate in HL, there is increased number of T-cells (CD4 and NKT subsets), decreased B-cells, and increased regulatory T-cells in comparision with reactive hyperplasia of lymph node; the tumor associated macrophages in HL are of prognostic importance. As it stands today, most of the cases of NHL and HL cases can be diagnosed based on cyto/histomorphology, immunocytochemistry, cytogenetic and molecular studies. However, there were some grey zone lymphomas, which do not exactly fall into either HL or NHL sub-types like ALCL and TCHRBCL. It appears that Hodgkin lymphoma and its pathogenesis is still in a stage of evolution and only future will tell when this turbulent phase will settle down.

INTRODUCTION

Hodgkin's disease (HD) is characterized by the presence of the typical, clonal malignant Hodgkin and Reed-Sternberg (HRS) cells in a hyperplastic background of normal reactive lymphocytes, plasma cells, histiocytes, neutrophils, eosinophils and stromal cells. [1] One hundred and eighty years have passed since the publication of an article in 1832 by Thomas Hodgkin (1798-1866) entitled "On some morbid appearances of the adsorbent glands and spleen," describing the post-mortem appearance of seven patients who had enlargements of these organs. [2] Thirty three years later, based on some 15 additional cases, Wilks published his article entitled "Cases of enlargement of the lymphatic glands and spleen, or, Hodgkin's disease with remarks," which ultimately named the disease after Thomas Hodgkin. [3] Carl von Sternberg in 1898 [4] and Dorothy Reed in 1902 [5] independently described the pathognomonic cell of Hodgkin's disease, presently called Hodgkin cell and Reed-Sternberg cell (HRS cells). The microenvironment of Hodgkin's disease is dominated by an extensive mixed and potentially inflammatory cellular infiltrate, and the HRS cells have several characteristics that are unusual for lymphoid tumor cells. [6] According to Cozen et al., [7] the histopathology and symptomatology of HD were reminiscent of chronic infectious granulomatous disease, but the untreated clinical course was that of a malignancy. However, molecular analysis has put all the speculations to rest and revealed that almost all cases of this disease are clonal B cell neoplasms; therefore the term Hodgkin's lymphoma instead of Hodgkin's disease was proposed in the new WHO classification [8] and in 2001, the World Health Organization (WHO) lymphoma classification system re-designated Hodgkin's disease to Hodgkin's lymphoma. [9] The present chapter is going to cover four and half decades, which accounts for exactly 25% of the entire history of Hodgkin's lymphoma and a period since the publication of the most widely used Rye classification [10] to the year 2011.

INCIDENCE AND FREQUENCY OF HL

As per a report one and half decade ago, the incidence of HD varied from about 0.5 per 100,000 person-years in parts of Asia to over 3 in parts of North America. [11] A recent publication also shows that Hodgkin's lymphoma (HL) is one of the most common lymphomas in the developed world, with an incidence of approximately three per 100,000 person-years. [12] Hodgkin's lymphoma comprises about 11% of all lymphomas in western countries and has a unique bimodal age-incidence shape. [13] During 1992-2001, the incidence of HL in USA was 2.67 per 100,000. [14] The crude incidence of HL in the European Union is 2.2 and mortality is 0.7 cases per 100,000 per year. [15] In Taiwan, the crude and age-adjusted rates of HL were 0.19-0.62 and 0.21-0.60 per 100,000 per year respectively, from year 1979 to 2002. [16] When the reported frequency of HL among all lymphoma cases from different countries of the world was analyzed (Table 1), [17-53] it ranged from 3.0% to 57.3% with a median of 17.8%. It was found that the frequency exceeded 10% in 5 (33.3%) among the 15 reports from Far-East countries [20-23, 30, 31, 34, 35, 39, 40, 43, 45, 47, 49, 53] and in 21 (95.5%) among 22 reports from the rest of the world [17-19, 24-29, 32, 33, 36-38, 41, 42, 44, 46, 48, 50-52] the difference being highly significant (p=0.00008). When the two groups were compared in respect of frequency exceeding 20%, none of reports from the Far-East countries had this feature as opposed to 15 (68.2%) from rest of the world (p=0.00002). When Sub-Saharan African countries were compared with rest of the non-Far-East countries of the world, it was observed that the frequency of HL exceeded 20% in 2 (28.6%) of the seven Sub-Saharan African countries [25, 26, 28, 29, 33, 37, 48] and 13 (86.7%) of the 15 among the other counties (p=0.01355). Thus, whereas Hodgkin's lymphoma is uncommon in the Far-East countries as compared to rest of the world, it is relatively uncommon in Sub-Saharan African countries.

Table 1. Frequency of Hodgkin's lymphoma versus of non-Hodgkin lymphoma in reports from various countries of the world. [17-53]

Authors (year)	Country	No of lymphomas	Frequency of HL versus NHL in %		
			HL	NHL	NOS
Bastien et al (1979) [17]	France	246	38.6	61.4	-
Radaszkiewicz (1980) [18]	Germany	800	22.9	77.1	-
Kelényi and Várbiró (1980) [19]	Hungary	383	18.0	78.9	3.1
Shimizu et al (1982) [20]	Japan	118	7.6	92.4	-
Ho et al (1984) [21]	China	294	9.2	90.8	-
Su et al (1985) [22]	Taiwan	104	8.7	86.5	4.8*
Calderon et al (1986) [23]	Philippines	434	18.0	82.0	-
Burla et al (1990) [24]	Germany	168	33.9	66.1	-

Authors (year)	Country	No of lymphomas	Frequency of HL versus NHL in %		
			HL	NHL	NOS
Okpala et al (1991) [25]	Nigeria	508	18.7	81.3	-
Walter et al (1991) [26]	Gabon	72	6.9	93.1	-
Ramani et al (1991) [27]	India	103	30.1	69.9	-
Obafunwa et and Akinsete (1992) [28]	Nigeria	167	32.3	67.7	-
Ngendahayo and Schmauz (1992) [29]	Rawnda	115	16.5	83.5	-
Ji and Li (1992) [30]	China	1082	9.4	90.4	-
Yang et al (1993) [31]	China	209	12.0	88.0	-
Dasgupta et al (1993) [32]	India	192	57.3	42.7	-
Cool and Bitter (1997) [33]	Kenya	73	17.8	82.2	-
Chai et al (1999) [34]	Malaysia	107	10.3	89.7	-
Chuang et al (2000) [35]	Taiwan	205	3.9	96.1	-
Castella et al (2001) [36]	UAE	208	40.9	59.1	-
Getachew (2001) [37]	Malawi	83	25.3	73.5	1.2
Naresh et al (2002) [38]	India	562	31.3	68.7	-
He et al (2003) [39]	China	370	3.0	97.0	-
Sukpanichnant (2004) [40]	Thailand	1983	7.9	92.1	-
Haddadin (2005) [41]	Jordan	347	21.6	78.4	-
Shivarov et al (2005) [42]	Bulgaria	790	24.6	73.3	2.2
Wang et al (2006) [43]	China	447	13.9	86.1	-
Hashemi-Bahremani et al (2007) [44]	Iran	385	28.1	71.9	-
Jeong et al (2007) [45]	Korea	507	6.7	93.3	-
Akhtar et al (2009) [46]	Saudi Arabia	385	30.4	65.2	4.4
Yoon et al (2010) [47]	Korea	5318	4.1	95.9	-
Mwakigonja et al (2010) [48]	Tanzania	158	15.2	84.8	-
Chen et al (2010) [49]	Taiwan	303	8.3	91.7	-
Chakrabarti et al (2010) [50]	India	124	38.7	61.3	-
Jayasekara et al (2010) [51]	Australia	28709	8.4	86.3	5.2
Yago et al (2011) [52]	Iraq	270	24.1	75.9	-
Yang et al (2011) [53]	China	6382	13.1	86.9	-

* Histiocytic malignancies.

Classifications of Hodgkin's Lymphoma

Hodgkin's lymphoma (HL), which was earlier known as Hodgkin disease (HD), is a malignant lymphoma whose unusual heterogeneous clinical, histologic, and epidemiologic features have suggested either a single disease entity with a complex host response or more than one possible distinct entity. [54] A comprehensive classification of HD was first proposed by Jackson and Parker in 1943, [55] which classified Hodgkin's disease into paragranuloma, granuloma and sarcoma subtypes; this classification was subsequently found to be clinically irrelevant because most of the patients belonged to ganuloma subtype with a huge variation in response to therapy and outcome. Lukes and Butler [56] suggested a histologic classification distinguishing 6 types of HD, viz., lymphocytic and/or histiocytic nodular, lymphocytic and/or histiocytic diffuse, nodular sclerosis, mixed cellularity, diffuse fibrosis and reticular based on a varying degrees of lymphocytic infiltration; this classification was simplified at the Rye symposium in 1965 and the number of histologic groups was reduced from 6 to 4 [10]: lymphoytic predominance, nodular sclerosis, mixed cellularity and lymphocytic depletion. The Rye classification was applied to routine histopathological and cytological diagnoses from mid-sixties to mid-nineties because of good clinicopathologic correlation and high reproducibility. In the mean time along with morphologic and clinical findings, studies on phenotypic, genotypic and molecular parameters threw new lights into the natural history of Hodgkin's disease. In view of these findings, HL was listed in the Revised European-American Lymphoma (REAL) classification, and subdivided into 2 main types [57]: nodular lymphocytic predominant nodular/diffuse HL and classic HL, the latter in turn was further divided into four subtypes: nodular sclerosis, mixed cellularity, lymphocyte rich diffuse (provisional) and lymphocyte depleted. This approach has been adopted by WHO classification of lymphomas, which promoted lymphocyte-rich classic HL from a provisional to an accepted entity. [9] Thus, the WHO classifications [9, 58] classified HL into nodular lymphocytic predominant HL (NLPHL) and classic HL (CHL), which in turn was divided into nodular sclerosis HL (grades 1 and 2), lymphocyte-rich HL (nodular and diffuse), mixed cellularity, lymphocytic depleted and unclassifiable HL.

Rye Classification

Nearly five decades ago Hodgkin's lymphoma, then known as Hodgkin's disease (HD), was classified into lymphocytic predominant (LP), mixed cellularity (MC), lymphocytic depletion (LD) and nodular sclerosis (NS) type. [10] Classification of Hodgkin's disease in FNA cytologic material was performed with satisfactory results following histologic criteria but nodular sclerosis type of HL, which is characterized by islands of neoplastic cells including a special type of R-S cells called lacunar cells and reactive cell components being surround by collagenous bands, was rarely sub-classified in cytologic preparations due to inherent difficulty in identifying these characteristics. [59] The sub-classification into LP, MC, and LD in histology as well as cytology depended on relative proportion of neoplastic HRS cells and reactive cellular components. Differential counts of HRS cells and reactive components in Hodgkin's disease by Das and Gupta [60] revealed significantly lower number of LP cases (6/26) with $\geq$1.5% HRS cells as compared to MC (32/39) and LD (9/9) subtypes (p<0.0001); and significantly lower number of MC (3/39) with ≥7.5% HRS cell compared to LD (7/9) subtypes (p<0.0001). Lymphocyte content exceeded 95% in 18 of 28 LP subtype, which was significantly higher than MC (8/39) and LD (0/9) subtypes (p<0.0001). In another report by Fuggle et al., [61] a significant difference was found between the mean percentages of eosinophil polymorphs between the subtypes of HD: LP (range 0-0.9%, mean 0.24%), NS (range 0-34.2%, mean 13.2%), MC (range 0-20.8%, mean 5.35%) and LD (range 8.2-31.9%, mean 22.6%). Crocker et al., [62] observed that the number of macrophage and macrophage-like cells as determined by α-naphthyl acetate esterase (ANAE)-positive staining in subtypes of HD was as follows: LP (1.8%-16%), NS (13.6%-22.1%), MC (6.5%-14.6%), and LD (39.8%-47.7%). Analysis of 33 reports on Rye classification from various countries (Table 2) [6, 7, 16, 25, 32, 44, 56, 63-88] revealed that the use of this classification continued well after the introduction of WHO classification. [6, 16, 44, 84-88] The range and median of the percentages of the four major subtypes of HL, viz., LP, NS, MC and LD were as follows: LP (range 3.1% to 27.3%, median10.0%), NS (range 2.6% to 74.4%, median 45.1%), MC (range 14.5% to 80.7%, median 35.0%) and LD (range 0% to 36%, median 6.2%), respectively. From the developed economies, [7, 56, 63-65, 69, 72, 73, 75, 81, 82, 84, 86] the median percentages for LP, NS, MC and LD subtypes were 10%, 58.5%, 26.0% and 2.6%, respectively. From the developing countries, [6, 16, 25, 32, 44, 66-68, 70, 71, 74, 76-80, 83, 85, 87, 88] the median percentages for LP, NS, MC and LD subtypes were 9.5%, 29.4%, 44.1% and 8.9%, respectively. In NS subtype, the frequency exceeded 50% in significantly higher number of reports from the developed (9 of 13, 69.2%) than developing countries (3 of 20, 15.0%, p= 0.00281). A reverse trend was observed when the reports with MC subtype exceeding 30% of cases were compared (23.1% of the reports in developed vs. 90.0% in the developing world, p=0.00016). However, there was no significant difference between the developed and developing countries in respect of LP and LD subtypes when the number of reports with frequency exceeding 10% were compared (p=1.0000, and =0.26346, respectively).

Application of immunohistochemical as well as other ancillary studies involving molecular parameters in HD in 1980s onwards threw light on true nature of HRS cell and nature of HL. Based on new findings, REAL/WHO classifications of HL were proposed. Not only difference between NLPHL and CHL started to become clear, NHL subtypes like ALCL and TCRBCL, which were earlier confused with HL could be separated from HL; and finally there was useful information on etiology of HL and the pathogenesis of HL could be understood with greater clarity.

Nature of HRS Cells

The histologic hallmark of Hodgkin's lymphoma is the presence of characteristic Hodgkin and Reed-Sternberg (HRS) cells in classical HL and so-called lymphocyte-predominant (LP) cells in nodular lymphocyte-predominant HL. [89] During 1950s and 1960s, Hodgkin cells and Reed-Sternberg (R-S) cells were traditionally believed to be abnormal reticulum cells. [90, 91] Rappaport [92] considered them to be of histiocytic origin on morphologic ground, although Dorfman [93] had failed to demonstrate lysosomal enzymes characteristic of macrophages in Reed-Sternberg cells. With the advent of immunological markers in 1970s, three candidates emerged as possible sources of HRS cells: T-lymphocytes, B-lymphocytes and macrophages; interdigitating reticulm cells and early progenitor myeloid cells subsequently joined the membership club of progenitor cells. A T-lymphocyte origin was proposed in a few studies. [94-96] In one of these reports, Binaminov and Ramot [95] demonstrated a T-cell abnormality rather than T-cell transformation. Payne et al. [97] also found that the T-cells cluster around the atypical cells but are not identical with them. Based on demonstration of cytoplasmic immunoglobulin (Ig) in R-S cells, a B-lymphocyte origin was also proposed. [98-100] However, some contemporary studies based on immunology and electron microscopy provided evidence against B-cell origin of R-S cells. Papadimitrou et al., [101] found that the intracytoplasmic immunoglobulin was polyclonal and the R-S cells contained both lysozyme and alpha-1-antitrypsin. Kadin et al. [102]concluded from their study that R-S cells did not synthesize immunoglobulin but ingested them from the extracellular environment. Along with Kadin and associates, [102] investigators in two other earlier studies favored macrophage as the malignant cell in Hodgkin's disease. [103, 104] According to Kaplan, [105] the capacity of Hodgkin cell and R-S cell for sustained proliferation in vitro, their aneuploidy and hetero-transplantability established their neoplastic character; further, the cell marker studies, phagocytic activity, positive staining reaction for nonspecific esterase and capacity to excrete lysozyme identify them as being derived from macrophages or other closely related cell of mononuclear phagocytic system, rather than from lymphocytes. In addition, the leaky membrane theory of Poppema et al. [106] and the theory of selective ingestion of Ig by Kadin et al., [102] supported the macrophage histogenesis. According to Maksem et al.,, [107] Hodgkin's disease was a malignant neoplasm that shared many histologic features with granulomatous disease; ultrastructurally, a close parallelism existed between the cells that typify granulomatous inflammation and Reed-Sternberg cells. It was the authors' contention [107] that the heterogeneity among R-S cells in all types of HD paralleled the diversity of the monocyte-macrophage system. However, during this period a report by Diehl et al., [108] based on long term cultures from tumor material revealed that in vitro, the cells have malignant characteristics that represent the in vivo H- and Rs cells but common immunological, functional and morphological assays did not characterize the in vitro cells to be a known cell type of lymphoid, myeloid or monocytoid tissue.

Experimental evidences suggested that multinucleated Reed-Sternberg cells with limited clonal growth capacity arose from mononuclear Hodgkin's cells by endomitosis. [109, 110] According to Drexler, [111] the mononuclear and polynuclear HRS cells are capable of DNA synthesis and nuclear division; the lack of cellular division leads to multinuclearity through the process of endomitosis. Farrell and Jarrett [12] showed that the HRS cells classically express the tumor necrosis factor receptor (TNFR) family member CD30 and the myeloid marker CD15; there may be aberrant expression of T-cell markers such as CD3, CD4 and granzyme B, and dendritic cell markers such as fascin and TARC (thymus activation-regulated chemokine, also known as CCL17) by HRS cells but the phenotype of HRS cell does not reveal B-cell origin. Markers of B lineage, such as CD20, CD19, CD79 and surface Ig, and transcription factors OCT2, BOB1 and PU1 are generally down-regulated in HRS cells, but B-cell specific transcription factor PAX5 is usually retained, albeit at low levels, and can be helpful in distinguishing CHL from T-cell lymphomas. On the other hand, LP cells express B-cell markers including CD20, CD79, PAX5, OCT2 and BOB1.

Table 2. Histological classification of Hodgkin's disease (HD) following Rye Classification [6, 7, 16, 25, 32, 44, 56, 63-88]

Authors (year)	Country	No of cases	Subtype of HD in percentages				
			LP	NS	MC	LD	UC
Lukes & Butler (1966) [56]	USA	377	16	40	26	18	-
Kadin et al (1971) [63]	USA	117	11	73	16	10	-
Gough (1970) [64]	UK	96	20	15	29	36	-
Farrer Brown et al (1971) [65]	UK	50	14	56	30	0	-
Wright (1973) [66]	Uganda	128	18	12	50	20	-
Mehrotra et al (1977) [67]	India	300	8	2.6	80.7	8.7	-
Das et al (1983) [68]	India	102	26.5	16.7	40.2	13.8	2.9
Petrella et al (1989) [69]	France	108	10.2	71.3	15.7	0.0	2.8
Liang et al (1989) [70]	Hong Kong	92	9.8	37.0	31.5	9.8	12
Soriano Rosas et al (1990) [71]	Mexico	422	5.9	19.7	41.5	6.2	26.8
Okpala et al (1991) [25]	Nigeria	95	18.9	17.9	45.3	17.9	-
Carde (1992) [72]	France	5096	6.3	63.9	24.6	1.9	3.2
Bernhards et al (1992) [73]	Germany	1045	3.0	63.2	18.9	0.8	14.2
Cozen et al (1992) [7]	USA	2492	10.0	50.0	32.0	8.0	-
Chang et al (1993) [74]	Peru	32	3.1	21.9	62.5	12.5	-
Dasgupta et al (1993) [32]	India	110	27.3	10.0	44.5	18.2	-
Medeiros and Greiner (1995) [75]	USA	9418	6.0	57.7	23.4	3.8	9.1
Rana et al (1995) [76]	India	104	16.3	16.3	57.7	9.7	-
De Souza et al (1997) [77]	Brazil	134	5.2	50.7	34.3	9.0	0.7
Peh et al (1997) [78]	Malaysia	100	15.0	41.0	40.0	3.0	1.0
Liu et al (1998) [79]	Taiwan	70	8.6	51.4	37.1	2.9	-
Monterroso et al (1998) [80]	Costa Rica	40	12.5	50.0	35.0	2.5	-
Mourad et al (1998) [81]	Canada	62	12.9	72.6	14.5	0	-
Enblad et al (1999) [82]	Sweden	117	4.3	74.4	17.9	2.6	0.9
Macák et al (2000) [83]	Czech Rep	142	9.2	45.1	43.7	2.1	-
Glavina-Durdov et al (2001) [84]	UK	100	8.0	48.0	37.0	7.0	-
De Oliveira et al (2002) [85]	Brazil	96	4.2	28.1	58.3	4.2	5.2
Krugmann et al (2003) [86]	Austria	119	5.9	58.8	32.8	2.5	-
Almasri and Khalidi (2004) [87]	Jordan	64	3.1	43.8	53.1	0.0	-
Vassalo et al (2005) [88]	Brazil	1025	4.9	69.3	21.2	4.7	-
Hashemi-Bahremani et al (2007) [44]	Iran	108	11.1	30.6	48.1	10.2	-
Wu et al (2008) [16]	Taiwan	133	12.8	45.1	28.6	2.3	11.3
Olu-Eddo and Omoti (2011) [6]	Nigeria	56	5.4	10.7	64.3	19.6	-

In an immunohistochemical study of 20 HD cases (5 NS, 12 MC, 3 LD), Wachi et al [112] observed that majority of RS-cells expressed CD30 and CD15, and some RS-cells could be of B-cell lineage since 7/20 cases consisting of 1 NS, 5 MC and 1 LD were CD20+. Schmid et al [113] performed immunohistochemistical and molecular analysis 55 patients with pre-treatment HD (45 NS, 10 MC) to determine the phenotype of H-RS cells; the H-RS cells were CD45- (100%), CD 30+ (100%), CD15+ (78%) and were reactive for at least one B-cell marker (CD19, CD20, CD22, CDw75, MB2) in 87% and a subpopulation of HRS cells were positive for T-cell marker (CD3, betaF1); all cases that expressed T-cell antigen were also reactive with at least one B-cell marker. The authors [113] were unable to confirm the previous reports of bcl-2 gene rearrangements in HD but the results strongly supported B-cell origin of H-RS cells. Zukerberg et al., [114] also demonstrated co-expression of B-cell marker CD20 and the granulocyte associated antigen CD15 by Reed-Sternberg cells, with some expressing CD20, some CD15, and others expressing both antigens. According to these authors, [114] cells co-expressing both CD15 and CD20 may represent an unstable intermediate in the process of antigen switching, and the possibility that antigen expression by neoplastic cells in a given case may modulate depending on the background infiltrate could explain the heterogeneity of immune-phenotype among cases of Hodgkin's disease. Immune-phenotypic analysis of H-RS cells by Drexler [111] also suggested a lymphoid cell expressing T- and/or B-cell associated markers and certain activated antigens while lacking immunological features of monocytes-macrophages or other lineages. In an immune-histochemical study of 92 CHL cases, the neoplastic cells were CD20+ in 12/84 (14.3%), CD15+ in 67/75 (89.3%), CD30+ in 75/77 (97.4%), and CD45RO in 0/75 (0.0%). [85] According to Chang et al., [115] there was no significant difference between Hodgkin's cells and R-S cells in respect of CD15 staining (82.8% vs. 74.6%), the common staining sites in the cell being Golgi region (71.1% vs. 61.9%) and cytoplasm (8.2% vs. 8.5%); similarly there was no significant difference between Hodgkin's and R-S cells in respect of CD30 staining (99.9% vs. 98.7%); the common sites in the cell being cytoplasm (69.2% vs. 63.6%) and ER-Golgi/cytoplasm (17.3% vs. 18.8%). According to Papadimitrou et al., [101] H-RS cells in 20% HD cases were CD57 positive, which were not of B-cell origin but may be related to natural killer (NK) or T-cells expressing CD57 antigens.

With the hypothesis that viral proteins may induce aberrant expression of cyclin A and lead to multinucleation in virus infected cells, Chang et al., [115] investigated whether Epstein-Barr virus (EBV) latent membrane protein-1 (LMP1) and cyclin A are involved in the morphogenesis of R-S cells, which represents the histologic hallmark for Hodgkin's lymphoma. These investigators [115]found that in LMP1+ and LMP1- HLs, multinucleated R-S cells aberrantly expressed cyclin A in cytoplasm, while the mononuclear Hodgkin cells expressed cyclin A predominantly in nuclei ($p<0.001$). No difference in expression of CD15, CD30 or CD99 in HL cells was found between the two groups. In vitro, EBV-LMP1 increased cytoplasmic cyclin A expression and multinucleation in an HL cell line. Therefore, the aberrant expression of cyclin A was thought to be commonly associated with RS cell morphologic features in HL, probably through LMP1 signaling or other similar mechanisms in EBV- cases. Bai, et al., [116] observed that EBV-positive cases, as demonstrated by the presence of EBER-1 and-2 RNA and LMP-1 protein expression, showed a significant reduction in expression on H-RS cells of T-cell lineage (CD3, $p<0.02$), B-cell lineage (CD20, $p<0.005$) and activation markers (EMA, $p<0.002$ and the 115D8 antigen, $p<0.001$) as compared to EBV-negative cases but no differences were found in the expression of CD15,

CD30, CD45RO, CD45RB, CDW75, or the MB2 antigen on H-RS cells in these two groups; these data suggested that EBV in H-RS cells was able to down regulate the expression of T-(CD3) and B-(CD20) cell lineage markers and lymphoid activation markers EMA and the 115D8 antigen.

The cellular origin of Hodgkin and Reed-Sternberg (HRS) cells, the neoplastic cells of classic Hodgkin's lymphoma (HL), resisted clarification until the second half 1990s. Siebert et al., [117]reported a case of HD (mixed cellularity) in which the H-RS cells expressed the characteristic markers CD15 and CD30; in addition they expressed CD19, CD20 and CD45/LCA and clonal rearrangement for Ig heavy chain gene was detected by Southern blot analysis. During the recent years, not only extensive phenotypical characterization HRS cells were performed, clonality of these cases has been demonstrated by cytogenetics and molecular genetics parameters. Immunophenotypical studies demonstrated frequent expression of "lymphoid activation markers" including CD15, CD25, CD30, CD40, CD54, CD70, CD71, CD80, CD86, and MHC class II and less frequent expression of T- or B-cell associated antigens by the neoplastic H-RS cells; the clonality of H-RS cells has been demonstrated by clonal EBV integration, clonal cytogenetic abnormalities including p53 mutations and clonal immunoglobulin rearrangements in some HD cases. [1]

According to Stein and Hummel, [118] one major obstacle to successful experimental investigations was the rarity of HRS cells in the tissue affected by HL; although the immunophenotypic studies pointed towards a B-cell origin of HRS cells in early 1980s, they were not definitive because of variable expression B-cell and/or T-cell antigens and the additional expression of markers typical for other lineages, especially dendritic cells, attempts to elucidate the cellular derivation by demonstrating the clonal rearrangements of the Ig gene or TCR genes in whole tissue extracts also remained inconclusive due inconsistent results. The extraction of single CD30+ HRS cells from immunostained frozen sections by means of hydraulic micromanipulation proved to be most suitable answer to these problems; using this method, monoclonal Ig gene rearrangements were detected in HRS cells in 95% of HL cases by Stein and Hummel [118] and their findings were summarized as follows: (1) Approximately 95% of classic HLs originate from B-cells; (2) the direct precursors of the HRS cells are germinal center B-cells; (3) the transforming event that causes HL leads to complete morphologic and immunophenotypical change of the HRS cell precursors; and (4) the HRS cell population of a given case exclusively arises from a single transformed cell and expands by clonal growth. The finding of Ig gene rearrangements in HRS cells in most cases of HD identified B cells as the precursors of HRS cells in most, if not all cases; furthermore, the presence and pattern of somatic mutations within the rearranged Ig genes showed that the HRS cells in classical (i.e. nodular sclerosis, mixed cellularity, and lymphocyte depletion HD) as well as lymphocyte predominant (LP) HD originated from germinal center (GC) B cells. [119] By molecular single cell analysis of Hodgkin and Reed-Sternberg (HRS) cells in Hodgkin's disease (HD), it could not only be shown that the HRS cells in classical as well as lymphocyte predominant (LP) HD represent clonal populations of mature B-cells but further information was obtained on their phenotypical differences; whereas HRS cells in classical HD appear to derive from crippled G B cells that lost the capacity to express antigen receptor, the precursors of the HRS cells in LP HD are mutating, antigen-selected GC B cells. [120] Tese findings were confirmed by many other studies in the years that followed. [110, 121, 122] According to Schmitz et al., [122] HRS cells have largely lost their B-cell phenotype and aberrantly express markers and transcriptional regulators of other hematolymphoid cell types; deregulation of multiple signaling pathways and downstream transcription factors, including receptor tyrosine kinases, nuclear factor-kappa B (NF-kappaB), and Janus kinase/signal transducer and activator of transcription (JAK/STAT) was a further hallmark of HRS cells.

Table 3. Histological classification of Hodgkin's disease (HD) following WHO classification [38, 42, 47, 48, 52, 53, 115, 138-147]

Authors (year)	Country	No of cases	Subtype of HL in percentages					
			NLPHL	CHLLR	CHLNS	CHLMC	CHLLD	CHLUC
LSGJP (2000) [138]	Japan	141	3.5	5.7	40.4	36.9	5.7	7.8
Naresh et al (2002) [38]	India	176	6.8	1.1	46.0	36.9	2.3	6.8 [†]
Makar et al (2003) [139]	Kuwait	134	6.7	3.0	37.3	45.5	3.0	4.5
De Matteo et al (2003) [140]	Argen-tina	173	2.9	6.9	38.7	48.6	2.9	-
Shivarov et al (2005) [42]	Bulgaria	194	1.0	1.0	64.4	23.2	5.7	4.6
Zhang et al (2006) [141]*	USA	42	0.0	6.1	39.4	36.4	12.1	6.1
Lee et al (2006) [142]	Taiwan	42	7.1	4.8	69.0	4.8	0.0	14.3
Keresztes et al (2006) [143]	Hungary	109	1.8	4.6	21.1	65.1	5.5	1.8
Al-Salam et al (2008) [144]	U.A.E.	88	10.2	1.1	45.5	31.8	4.5	6.8
Hudnall et al (2008) [145]	USA	59	8.5	3.4	69.5	15.3	3.4	-
Fong et al (2009) [146]	Austria	158	6.3	2.5	60.1	27.8	-	3.2
Chang et al (2009) [115]	Taiwan	34	2.9	11.8	67.6	14.7	0.0	2.9
Trankov e al (2010) [147]	Switze-rland	105**	-	2.9	57.1	30.5	1.9	7.6
Mwakigonja et al (2010) [48]	Tanzania	24	8.3	12.5	25.0	45.8	8.3	-
Yoon et al (2010) [47]	Korea	219	3.7	3.2	55.7	25.6	4.1	7.8
Yago et al (2011) [52]	Iraq	65	4.6	1.5	47.7	36.9	9.2	-
Yang et al (2011) [53]	China	833	4.2	4.2	17.4	72.7	1.4	-

* FNA-based study.** Only CHL cases included. [†]Included 4.0% CHL NOS and 2.8% UC HL. LSGJP= Lymphoma Study Group of Japanese Pathologists.

The above developments have been summarized by Farrell and Jarrett [12] in the following lines: microdissection coupled with analysis of immunoglobulin genes revealed that HRS cells are usually clonal B-cells. HRS cells, from nearly all CHL cases, and LP cells have detectable rearrangements of Ig heavy and/or light chain genes, confirming a B-cell origin and, in any given case, the rearrangements are identical, proving the clonal nature of the disease. Furthermore, the Ig variable (IgV) gene regions show evidence of somatic hypermutation, revealing a germinal centre (GC) or post-GC origin. In LP cells intraclonal IgV gene diversity is observed, indicating ongoing somatic hypermutation, whereas HRS cells show identical somatic hypermutation consistent with a later stage of B-cell differentiation, 'crippling' mutations, resulting in non-functioal Ig genes, are observed in around 25% of CHL cases. Rarely (<2%), HRS cells harbor rearranged T cell receptor genes, suggesting a T-cell origin in a small minority of cases.

Nature of Hodgkin's Lymphoma

Two findings, in particular, make HL a unique malignant hematopoietic disease: first, the malignant mononucleated Hodgkin- and the multinucleated Reed-Sternberg (HRS) cells represent only a small fraction of cells (about 1% cells in tumor tissue) in the affected lymph nodes and are embedded in an infiltrate of reactive hematopoietic cells, composed of B- and T-lymphocytes, eosinophils, and plasma cells among others, and second, the HRS cells do not display a phenotype that can be assigned to a defined hematopoietic cell type. [123] One of the earliest reports on Hodgkin's lymphoma involving immunohistochemical parameters was undertaken by Aisenberg and Wilkes [124] to study the lymphocyte population in Hodgkin's disease (HD) and reactive hyperplasia (RH) using a panel of 10 monoclonal antibodies and rosetting techniques; in both Hodgkin's disease and hyperplasia, 60%-70% of the cells were T lymphocytes and approximately 80% of these were inducer/helper subset and 20% cytotoxic/suppressor subset. The most prominent difference between HD and RH was explained by greater affinity of the sheep cell receptor on the surface of T lymphocyte of HD as compared to RH. Facchetti et al., [125] observed that plasmacytoid monocytes (so called plasmacytoid T-cells) were one of the monocyte-derived cells that contributed to the cellular reaction in HD (LP, NS and MC); they occurred at the periphery of lymphoid aggregates which mimicked the composite nodules of reactive lymph node but contained RS-cell and its variants.

In the past, various possibilities put forth regarding nature of Hodgkin's disease. Before 1950s the nature of Hodgkin's disease was thought to be inflammatory, [4, 5, 126] neoplastic [127-129] and an intermediate state between the two. [3, 130] A fourth possibility was put forth by Kaplan and Smithers, [131] who suggested that Hodgkin's disease might represent an autoimmune process. During late 1960s and 1970s, evidence in favor of neoplastic nature of Hodgkin's disease emerged. Studies involving incorporation of tritiated thymidine into DNA proved that Hodgkin cells and Reed-Sternberg cells were the proliferating cells. [132-134] Kaplan and Gartner [103]not only demonstrated incorporation of tritiated thymidine in DNA of Hodgkin cells and R-S cells but also observed binucleated mitotic figures, which proved that R-S cells arise by nuclear replication rather than by cell fusion. Aneuploidy of Hodgkin's cells was demonstrated [135, 136] and their clonal derivation was described, thus fulfilling two of the most fundamental attributes of neoplasia. According to Gruss and Kadin, [1] the neoplastic nature of HD is based on aggressive clinical progression, presence of the proliferating and atypical H-RS cells, aneuploidy and cellular clonality; the histopathological presentation and characteristic histopathological features of HD correlates with the unbalanced production of multiple cytoknes and thus, HD is defined as a tumor of cytokine-producing cells in which the proportion of malignant H-RS cells to reactive cellular components and fibrosis is dependent on the production of particular cytokines and this allows sub-typing of HD cases.

WHO Classification of Hodgkin's Lymphoma

New discoveries on nature of Hodgkin's disease and its pathognomonic neoplastic cells led to formulation of new classifications of Hodgkin's disease under auspices REAL/WHO. [137] As discussed earlier Hodgkin's disease was renamed Hodgkin's lymphoma and classified under WHO classification of hematopoietic neoplasms [9, 58] into two broad categories, viz., nodular lymphocytic predominance Hodgkin's lymphoma (NLPHL) and classical Hodgkin's lymphoma (CHL); CHL in turn under WHO classification, was classified into four subtypes: lymphocyte-rich (LRCHL), nodular sclerosis (NSCHL), mixed cellularity (MCCHL) and lymphocyte depletion (LDCHL), with a wide geographical variation in frequency (Table 3). [38, 42, 47, 48, 52, 53, 115, 138-147] However, unlike the Rye classification, no definite geographical trend was observed in distribution of subtypes, which may be due to smaller number of studies. The range and median values for frequency of various subtypes were as follows: NLPHL (0.0% to 10.2%, 4.2%), LRCHL (1.0% to 12.5%, 3.4%), NSCHL (17.4% to 69.5%, 46.0%), MCCHL (4.8% to 72.7%, 36.4%), LDCHL (0.0%-12.1%, 3.4%) and UCCHL (0.0% to 14.3%, 4.5%), respectively. Although the frequency of reports having >50%NSCHL was more, and >5% NLPHL, >5% LRCHL, >30% MCCHL, >5% LDCHL was less in the Far-East countries as compared to rest of the world, the difference was not significant (p=0.28006 to =1.00000).

Nodular Lymphocytic Predominant Hodgkin's Lymphoma (NLPHL)

NLPHL is a distinct HL subtype composed of few neoplastic lymphocyte predominant (LP) cells in a background of reactive small B and T cells. [148] Initial description of NLPHL was one characterized by a nodular, or nodular and diffuse proliferation of scattered and large neoplastic cells (lymphocytic and/or histiocytic [L&H] cells or "popcorn" cells) in large spherical mesh-works of follicular dendritic cells (FDCs) filled with non-neoplastic small lymphocytes, mainly of B-cell type. [149] At present the term lymphocytic predominant (LP) cell has replaced the "L&H" or "popcorn" cell. The recent description of NLPHL by Mani and Jaffe [150] is as follows: The LP cell has a polylobated nucleus with finely dispersed chromatin and small, usually basophilic nucleoli, and relatively sparse cytoplasm, which is immunohistochemially CD15-, CD30- (rare weak+), CD20+, CD79a+, CD45+, J-chain+, OCT+, BOB1+, PU1+, PAX+, and EBV-. Background shows small lymphocytes in a nodular or nodular and diffuse pattern (with focal presence of nodular pattern at least). The small lymphocytes in the background are small B-cells with a mantle cell phenotype (IgD+, IgM-). There are expanded mesh-works of FDC, as seen by CD21 immunostain. Epithelioid histiocytes are present in varying numbers.

Classical Hodgkin's Lymphoma (CHL)

The HRS cells of CHL possess single to multilobated nuclei with peripherally condensed chromatin, large and often eosinophilic nucleoli and abundant cytoplasm; the HRS cells are CD15+ (membrane and/or Golgi region), CD30+ (membrane and/or Golgi region), CD20 variable + (positive in 30-40% cases), CD79a- to variable weak+, CD45-, J-chain-, OCT-2- (often), BOB1- (often), PU1-, PAX5+ (weak), and EBV+ (variable). [150] The histopathological features of four subtypes of CHL are as follows:

- LRCHL: By definition, lymphocyte-rich CHL is a diffuse tumor with relatively infrequently R-S cells, which are of classic type, However, a nodular or follicular variant occurs, in which classical HRS cells are few in number and can be seen in marginal/mantle zone around regressed GCs with dense FDC meshwork. Aggregates of epithelioid histiocytes may be present, but eosinophils and neutrophils are rare.
- NSCHL: Capsular fibrosis and broad collagen bands, which are often perivascular, characterize this subtype; lacunar cells (a special type of HRS cells) and mummified cells are important features. Grade I and II differ in number of HRS cells and necrosis is a feature of grade II.
- MCCHL: There is diffuse lymph node effacement with numerous HRS cells and a mixed inflammatory background with lymphocytes, eosinophils, plasma cells and histiocytes. Granulomas may be present.
- LDCHL: Whereas diffuse fibrosis variant has a hypo-cellular background, abundant disorderly arranged non-birefringent fibrosis, abundant histiocytes but fewer lymphocytes; the reticular variant shows numerous HRS cells with bizarre cytological features.

Lymphocyte depleted classical Hodgkin lymphoma (LDCHL) is a vanishing category of classical. Hodgkin lymphoma, accounts for approximately <1% of all cases in the most modern series. [151]

DIFFERENCE BETWEEN NLPHL AND CHL

Pinkus and Said [152] observed that the L&H variant of R-S cells detected in LPHL, nodular were strongly immunoreactive for leukocyte common antigen and B-cell-specific antigens but uniformly non-reactive to Leu-1, granulocyte-related antigen; on the other hand the other types of R-S cells detected in NS, MC, and LD subtypes were strongly reactive for Leu-1 but non-reactive or rarely positive for LCA and negative for pan-B-cell monoclonal antibodies. According to these authors, [152] the L&H variants of RS-cells represent a distinct type of transformed cells, possibly of B-cell origin, and do not share a common lineage with other type of R-S cells; therefore LPHL, nodular may represent a distinct entity. Subsequently this distinct entity was named nodular lymphocytic predominant Hodgkin's disease (NLPHD). In all cases of NLPHD, the L&H cells were L26 positive. Other variants of RS cells, e.g., lacunar, mononuclear and diagnostic forms, which were present in NS, MC and LD subtypes, L26 positivity was noticed in <5% cells in 87% cases and in the remaining cases a larger proportion of these cells expressed L26. [153] Poppema [154] reported on the immunophenotype of nonneoplastic, small lymphocytes associated with HL; the T-cells in NLPHL, nodular sclerosing Hodgkin's lymphoma (NSHL) and mixed cellular Hodgkin's lymphoma (MCHL) displayed an activated CD4+ immunophenotype. However, the T-lymphocytes in NLPHL differed from NSHL and MCHL in that they showed reactivity for Leu 7 (CD57). Moreover, T-cells were found surrounding the R-S cells and variants in all three forms of HL but in only NLPHL these T-cells demonstrated CD57 reactivity. Poppema [154] suggested that CD57 immunoreactivity may be a helpful criterion for diagnosis of NLPHL. In an attempt to test the above hypothesis, Kamel et al., [155] used an image analysis system and found that the average of CD57 reactivity was 18.9% of small lymphocytes in NLPHL, 3.9% in NSHL, 4.3% in TCRBCL and 2.1% in follicular lymphoma. Further, the CD57+ lymphocytes showed a distinctive pattern in NLPHL, forming a ring of cells around the large L&H cells. According to Montes-Moreno, [156]the characteristic lymphocyte-predominant (LP) cells of NLPHL exhibit a germinal center (GC) phenotype profile with expression of GC markers such as BCL6, GCET1 and LMO2, together with expression of transcriptional factors related to a sustained B cell program such as OCT2 and BOB1. Interestingly, the GC-related profile is seen not only in LP cells but also in the surrounding T cells, which characteristically create a rosette-like pattern typical of NLPHL. These rosetting T-cells have a follicular T-cell phenotype with expression of CD3/CD4/CD57, bcl6, PD1 and, interestingly, CXCL13, a chemokine that is known to induce B-cell homing to lymphoid follicles and that plays a role in the T cell-dependent B cell affinity maturation process. These observations suggest that NLPHL is characterized by a GC phenotype in both LP and surrounding T-cells. This combination is not found in classical HL (CHL), with the exception of lymphocyte-rich CHL, which has a profile intermediate between NLPHL and CHL with overexpression of B-cell transcription program markers and the presence of follicular T-cell background in a substantial proportion of cases. This is not the case of other types of CHL in which the B cell program and the germinal center microenvironment is lost.

As it stands today, the NLPHL can be distinguished from CHL based on clinical, morphological, immunophenotypical and genetic features. The growth pattern in NLPHL is at least in part nodular mostly and diffuse pattern is very rare; the neoplastic cells are LP cells (L&H cells or popcorn cells) with nuclei resemble those of centroblasts having polylobular profile, finely dispersed chromatin and small nucleoli adjacent to nuclear membrane. The immunophenotype of the neoplastic cells in NLPHL are CD45+, CD20+, CD22+, CD79a+, J chain±, EMA±, CD15- and CD30- or weak+. The lymph node in CHL is largely effaced although remnants of follicle can be detected in some cases. In CHL, the typical Hodgkin's and Reed-Sternberg cells can be easily detected and can be associated with peculiar variants and the immunophenotype of H&RS cells is CD30+ (98%), CD15+ (80%), CD45-, EMA-, CD20+ (30%-40%) and CD79a (even less frequently); one or more T-cell markers are seen in a minority of H&RS cells in some cases. More specifically, the nodular lymphocyte-rich variant of classical Hodgkin lymphoma (CHL), can be differentiated NLPHL from based on immunophenotype. In contrast to CHL, tumor cells of NLPHL do not express CD30 and CD15, but they are positive for B-cell markers (CD20, CD79a), immunoglobulins, J chain, and EMA. [149] The B-cell phenotype and genetic features of NLPHL, exhibiting clonally rearranged immunoglobulin genes with ongoing mutations, [157, 158] indicate its close relationship to B-cell non-Hodgkin lymphomas. [9, 159]

DIFFERENTIAL DIAGNOSIS OF HODGKIN'S LYMPHOMA

When the Rye classification on Hodgkin's disease was formulated in 1966, [10] it was regarded by many as a formidable classification since the diagnostic criteria for Hodgkin's disease were very sound, which could not be challenged easily. During 1970s, understanding of the nature of cells in the formation of non-Hodgkin's lymphoma (NHL) led to the emergence of a number of classifications and a wide range of controversies was associated with it. Unlike non-Hodgkin's lymphoma, the fortress of Hodgkin's lymphoma seemed invincible in seventies through eighties into early nineties. However, as seen in table 1, 1.2% to 5.2% cases were unclassified as lymphomas other than HL and NHL with a median of 3.8% in six studies. [19, 22, 37, 42, 46, 51] When Hodgkin's disease were classified as per Rye classification, in 12 of the 33 studies (Table 2), 0.7% to 26.8% HL cases were also unclassified. [16, 69-73, 75, 77, 78, 82, 85] This is again highlighted in WHO classification (Table 3), wherein 12 out of 17 studies had 1.8% to 14.3% cases were unclassified HL. [38, 42, 47, 115, 138, 139, 141-144, 146, 147] These findings indicate that there were cases in which decision between NHL and HL was difficult or not possible, and also cases in which classifying HL into subtypes based not only on morphological features but even with all ancillary parameters was difficult. In earlier reports, the so called pathognomonic HRS cells or HRS-like cells were reported not only in benign lymphoproliferative conditions like reactive lymphoid hyperplasia and infectious mononucleosis, but some of nonHodgkin lymphoma subtypes, e.g., chronic lymphocytic leukemia, mycosis fungoides, Burkitt's lymphoma, lymphoepithelioid lymphoma and immunoblastic lymphoma, and non-lymphoid malignancies like metastatic carcinoma, melanoma, sarcoma and germ cell tumors revealed presence of RS-like cells. [160-162] The application of T-cell and B-cell lymphoid markers for immunophenotyping and/or genetic probe methods have further confirmed the suspicion of pathologists that morphologic similarities do exist between HD, and some pleomorphic T-cell lymphomas, [163]T-cell-rich B-cell lymphoma (TCRBCL) [164] and anaplastic large cell lymphoma (ALCL). [165]Review of HL cases in some of the studies yielded NHL ranging from 1.9% to 14.3% with a median of 10.4%.[69, 72, 166, 167].

According to Harris, [168] the immunophenotype and genetic features are useful in the classification of HL and in distinguishing HL from two recently described, aggressive lymphomas that were in the past often diagnosed as HL, i.e., anaplastic large-cell lymphoma, T-cell type, and T-cell/histiocyte-rich large B-cell lymphoma. Elgin et al., [169] felt that immunoperoxidase markers are useful and often essential in distinguishing among lymphocytic predominant Hodgkin's lymphoma, T-cell-rich B-cell lymphoma, and lymphocyte-rich classical Hodgkin's lymphoma; however, it is becoming increasingly clear that these "entities" are closely related clonal B-lineage neoplasms that may inter-transform and/or coexist. Das et al., [170] reported that ALCL and TCRBCL are the most common

NHL subtypes to be confused with HL but other entities like pleomorphic T-cell lymphomas and some large B-cell lymphomas may give rise to the diagnostic difficulties. This will be apparent from the few other reported studies in yester years. In a study of 2 NPHL and 43 CHL cases by Liu et al.,, [170] the NLPHL cases were CD20+, CD15-, CD30-; CD57+ cells and small B-lymphocytes were predominant cells in the background infiltration; diagnostic RS cells and other tumor cells in 43 CHL cases were positive for CD30 (100%), CD15 (81%), and CD20 (7%). Whereas six TCRBCL cases were negative for CD15 and CD30, two ALCL cases were CD30+, ALK1+, CD3+, CD15- and CD20-. The reactive inflammatory cell infiltration present in CHL cases were rich in TIA1+ cytotoxic lymphocytes but CD57+ cells were rarely encountered. The comparative genomic hybridization (CGH) profiles of THCRBCL and NLPHL showed some common and several distinct features, in particular with respect to the number of genomic imbalances (average of 4.7 in T/HRBCL versus 10.8 in LPHL) and their distribution (usually 1 to 5 in T/HRBCL versus 6 to 22 in LPHL). [171]Thus, T/HRBCL constitutes a separate lymphoma entity, possibly originating from the same precursor cell as LPHL. In a cyto-histologic study of 15 ALCL and 48 HL cases, Mourad et al., [172] observed an immunohistochemical profile of CD15+, CD30+ and CD45- pattern in HL, and CD15-, CD30+ and CD45+ in ALCL cases; immunostaining with ALK antibody revealed positive reaction in 3 of 8 ALCL cases. As per a review of literature by Marafioti et al., [173] the neoplastic cells of TCRBCL were LSP-1 positive and PU.1 negative, whereas the L&H cells of lymphocyte predominance HL were mostly LSP-1 negative, with variable PU.1 expression; however, the two markers did not distinguish between TCRBCL and lymphocyte-rich classical HL. The transcription factor PU.1 is down-regulated in TCRBCL compared with lymphocyte predominant HL; PU.1 regulates the transcription of genes relevant to the development of B-cells, macrophages and myeloid cells. Leukocyte-specific phosphoprotein (LSP1) is present in the neoplastic cells of most large B-cell lymphomas, but usually absent in lymphocyte-predominant HL.

Etiology of HL: Role of Epstein Barr Virus (EBV) and Other Viral Agents

EBV plays an important role in several neoplasms, in particular, African endemic Burkitt's lymphoma and Chinese nasopharyngeal carcinoma in south-east Asia; other diseases such as Hodgkin's disease, some NHL, gastric cancer and esophageal cancer have some relationship with EBV. [85, 174] According to Jarrett, [175] EBV is an extremely efficient transforming agent and when EBV infects B-cells in vitro, six EBNA (EBNA-6) proteins (EBNA 1, 2, 3a, 3b, 3c and LP) are expressed alongside three membrane proteins (LMP1, LMP2A and LMP2B). Recent molecular studies provide support for the idea that EBV is involved in the pathogenesis of HD. EBV genomes are consistently found in a proportion of tumor biopsies, EBV infected cells are clonal; not only the EBV genomes have been localized to Reed Sternberg cells, EBV latent gene products are expressed in R-S cells. [176] Furthermore, since majority of samples from patients aged greater than 50 years and less than 15 years are fund to be EBV positive, it is suggested that EBV plays a role in HD in children and older adults but that other agents, possibly other viruses, are involved in young adults. [176]In the Chinese population, tumor cells of 39% of CHL patients were EBV+ and this was significantly associated with male sex, mixed cellular subtype, young age (<20y). [177] A review by Chang et al., [74] showed that patients with HD have abnormally high levels of antibodies against EBV antigens and EBV-associated infectious mononucleosis patients have an increased risk of HD over control populations. A review by Makar et al., [139]of 14 studies from Arabian Gulf and Middle East region, Asia, North America and Western Europe and Africa and South America revealed EBV positivity in 382/776 (49.2%) cases; the positivity in LP, NS, MC, LD and unclassifiable cases was 10/57 (17.5%), 168/447 (37.6%), 201/276 (72.8%), 22/32 (68.8%), and 3/8 (37.5%), respectively. Testing of EBV within the RS and Hodgkin cells was carried out in childhood Hodgkin's lymphoma in 10 different countries. The proportion of LMP1 positive cases varied significantly, being 50% of cases from UK, South Africa, Egypt, and Jordan, 60% from UAE, 70% from Australia, 81% from Costa Rica, 88% from Iran, 90% from Greece, and 100% of the 56 cases from Kenya. [178] Peh et al., [78] found that in younger (<15 years) patients, 93% were positive for EBV and in older patients 52% were positive. According to Liu et al, [79] the association of EBV with HL is intimately related to socioeconomic status with high prevalence in developing countries and low prevalence in developed countries; in a study of 70 HL cases from Taiwan overall EBV positivity was 44 (62.9%). A comparative study of 33 HD cases from Kenya and 31 cases from Nagasaki, Japan revealed EBER positivity by ISH in 79% in Kenya and 59% in Nagasaki. [174] The frequency of EBV positivity by LMP-1 by IHC and EBER by ISH from 14 different studies (11 on Rye classification and 3 based on WHO classification of HL) has been depicted in table 4. [74, 78-83, 85-87, 115, 139, 143, 144]Overall EBV positivity ranged from 26.1%to 93.8%, with a median 46.8%. Under Rye classification, the range and median of EBV positivity for the subtypes were as follows: LP (0%-100%, 0%), NS (15%-100%, 29.6%), MC (38.1%-100%, 74.2%) and LD (14%-100%, 50.0%), respectively. [74, 78-83, 85-87, 143]In WHO classification, the range and median of EBV positivity in various subtypes were as follows: NLPHL (0%-2%, 2%), LRCHL (25%-100%, 50%), NSCHL (27.3%-478%, 34.2%), MCCHL (52.9%-100%, 79.2%) and LDCHL (50%-100%, 75%), respectively. [115, 139, 144]

Benharroch et al., [179] in a cohort of 154 HD patients detected positive immunostaining for at least two anti-measles antibodies in 82 (54.3%); while immunostaining for EBV LMP-1 protein was positive in 46 (31.1%); reverse transcriptase-PCR and ISH for measles RNA were positive in 7 and 10 of 28 patients, respectively. In setting of high prevalence HIV infection in South Africa, 2225 new cases of lymphoproliferative disorders were diagnosed during 2007-2009 as compared with 1897 cases diagnosed during 2004-2006; [180] a significant increase in both high-grade B-cell lymphomas and Hodgkin's lymphoma was documented during 2007-2009 and this was associated with a statistically significant increase in HIV prevalence in those tested (from 44.3% in 2004-2006 to 62.0% in 2007-2009).

PHENOTYPIC, GENOMIC AND MOLECULAR DEFECTS IN HRS CELLS: THE SIGNIFICANCE

Hodgkin's lymphomas belong to the most curable neoplasti diseases in adults; about 80% of patients in all anatomical stages and of all histological subtypes can be cured with modern treatment strategies. [181] It has been observed since long that patients with lymphocyte depletion, NOS, and mixed cellularity subtype of HL have a significantly worse prognoses compared to patients who had nodular sclerosis, whereas patients who had lymphocytic predominance had the best prognosis. [182] Using three marker (CD15, CD20 and CD30) in 1751 classical (non-lymphocytic predominant) HD cases Von Wasielewsky et al., [183] found 83% with classical phenotype (CD15+, CD30+, CD20-); 12% lacked CD15 positivity (CD15-, CD30+, CD20-) and 5% showed other combinations. According to these authors, [183] clinical follow-up of 1286 cases revealed significant difference for freedom from treatment failure (p=0.0022) and overall survival (p=0.0001) between cases with classical immunophenotype and those with CD15- (CD30+, CD20-); multivariate Cox regression analysis showed that lack of CD15 expression in classical HD is an independent negative prognostic factor for relapse (p=0.022) and survival (p= 0.0035). In a study 110 HD patients by Smolewski et al., [184] 69 obtained complete remission (CR) after first-line treatment and 41 did not respond. Evaluating apoptosis by TUNEL technique (TdT-mediated dUTP nick end labeling), these authors [184] found positive TUNEL reaction in 43 patients with apoptotic index (AI) varying between 10% and 60%; in the remaining 57 patients AI of H-RS cells was <10%; the mean AI in non-responding patients was significantly higher than in CR group (p=0.015); the high frequency of AI was also negatively correlated with the progression free survival time (p=0.031) and the overall survival (p=0.042).

Quite a few immunophenotypic and molecular studies on the prognosis of HL are based on Epstein Barr virus (EBV). Two pathogenic mechanisms are probably influenced by the presence of EBV in the H-RS cells: resistance of the H-RS cells to apoptosis; and escape of H-RS cells from a cytotoxic T lymphocyte immune response; [185]latent membrane protein-1 (LMP-1) is most likely the EBV-encoded protein responsible for this putative EBV-mediated pathogenic effect. Oudejans et al., [185]found that with the use of conventional therapy regimens, the presence of EBV bears little influence on clinical presentation and treatment outcome of HD. However, the difference in regulation of both apoptosis and immune escape mechanisms between EBV+ and EBV- cases may be important determinants of the success of immune therapy to treat Hodgkin's disease. Krugmann et al., [86] observed that patients with EBV-associated classical HL were predominantly mixed cellular type; were more frequent in male patients, in those above 45 years of age, in Stage III and IV disease, and in patients with B-symptoms; showed a significantly longer mean time of first relapse of 99 months as compared with 49 months for EBV-negative cases (p<0.02). However, overall survival did not correlate with EBV-association. Thus, the presence of EBV has a beneficial effect on the length of failure-free survival despite the higher frequency of risk factors such as higher tumor stage or advanced age. According to Keegan et al., [186] EBV in HL cells has been considered a prognostic marker for this heterogeneous disease, but studies have yielded mixed findings, likely because of selected patients series and failure to acknowledge the effect of age. In a study by these authors, [186] EBV presence in children less than 15 years old was suggestively associated with favorable survival (p=0.07); in adults aged 15 to 44 years, EBV did not affect HL outcome, although a protective effect was suggested; in older adults (45 to 96 years), EBV presence nearly doubled the risk of overall and HL-specific mortality but only with nodular sclerosis subtype. Thus, EBV tumor presence is associated with better survival in young patients in HL and poorer survival in older patients with NS HL.

Table 4. Epstein-Barr virus (EBV) studies in Hodgkin's disease/lymphoma as per Rye and WHO classification [74, 78-83, 85-87, 115, 139, 143, 144]

Author and year	Country	No of cases studied		+vity in %	EBV +vity in subtypes of HL in percentages					
		Ove-rall	LMP1(L) /EBER (E)		NLP	LP/ LR*	NS	MC	LD	UC
Chang et al, 1993 [74]	Peru		LMP: 25	78.1		0	77.3	90.0	25.0	-
			EBER: 30	93.8		100	100	100	50.0	-
Peh et al, 1997 [78]	Malaysia	81		50.6		0	22.2	86.4	50.0	100
Monterosso et al, 1998 [80]	Costa Rica		LMP: 40	40.0		0	15.0	85.7	100	-
Liu et al, 1998 [79]	Taiwan	70		62.9		16.7	63.9	69.2	100	-
Mourad et al, 1998 [81]	Saudi Arabia	62		46.8		0	46.7	88.9	-	
Enblad et al, 1999 [82]	Sweden	117		27.4		20.	23.0	38.1	100	0
Macák et al, 2000 [83]	Czech Republic	142		33.1		38.5	25.0	38.7	66.7	-
De Oliveira et al, 2002 [85]	Brazil	96		63.5		0	29.6	83.9	25.0	100
Krugmann et al, 2003 [86]	Austria		LMP: 119	26.1		0	21.4	38.5	33.3	-
			EBER: 107	29.0		0	23.4	44.1	33.3	-
Almasri and Khalidi, 2004 [87]	Jordan	64		46.9		0	28.6	64.7	-	-
Keresztes et al, 2006 [143]	Hungary	109		43.1		-	34.8	49.3	-	-
Makar et al, 2003 [139]	Kuwait	107*		56.1	2	50.0	34.2	79.2	100	33.3
Al-Salam et al, 2008 [144]	UAE	45*		37.8	0	100	27.3	52.9	50.0	-
Chang et al, 2009 [115]	Taiwan	34*	LMP: 13	38.2						
			EBER: 18	52.9	0	25.0	47.8	100	-	100

* These studies were based on WHO classification and LP subtype of Rye classification was replaced with lymphocyte-rich (LR) subtype and nodular lymphocyte predominant (NLP) HL was a separate entity from CHL.

SIGNIFICANCE OF MICROENVIRONMENT IN HL

In a study by Von Wasielewski et al, [187] prominent eosinophilia was detected 38% of HL cases overall, which differed among histologic subtypes: LP (0%), LRCHL (14%), NS1CHL (40%), NS2CHL (55%), MCCHL (43%) and LDCHL (54%). In a multivariate analysis, tissue eosinophilia proved to be the strongest prognostic factor (indicating poor prognosis) for freedom of treatment failure (P<0.001) and overall survival (P<0.001), and this effect was most significant among NSCHL, especially NS1CHL cases, however, in MCCHL no significant effect of eosinophilia on survival could be demonstrated. [187] Eosinophils secrete CD30 ligand that is capable of binding to CD30 positive HRS cells, which in turn leads to activation of TRAF2, followed by NF-κB and thereby neoplastic proliferation and apoptosis protection of HRS cells. With the possibility that eosinophils are only passive indicators of unknown prognostic determinants, it may be concluded that the positive clinical outcome of eosinophilia-negative NSCHL cases could be due to lower NF-κB activity. Applying a cutoff score of >0.82% CD68+ tumor macrophages, Tzankov et al., [147] observed worse overall survival in increased number of CHL cases (mean 185 months, median 192 months) compared to cases with lower number (mean 285 months, median not reached); eleven of 62 CHL patients with ≤0.82% tumor macrophages died, compared to 19 of 43 with >0.82% (p<0.001). Expression of markers for various tumor associated macrophages (TAMs), viz., CD68, HLA-DR, CD163, HLA-DR/CD68 (M1) and CD163/CD68 (M2) were immunohistochemically studied by Zaki et al., [188] in classical HL. Number of CD163+ cells and M2+ cells was significantly correlated with shorter overall survival (p<0.05), while it was marginally significant for CD68+ cells (p=0.0827). While confined to MC subtype, number of M1+ cells correlated with favorable prognosis (p<0.05), while M2 did not (p=0.7). At multivariate analysis, number of CD63+ cells, M2+ cells, and age were independent factors for poor overall survival (p=0.03, =0.02, and =0.01, respectively). Thus, CD163+ cells and M2+ cells might work as tumor promoter cells in CHL and M1+ cells might be tumor suppressive in MC subtype. Sohani et al., [148] observed 11 NLPHL in which, in addition to typical B-cell-rich nodules containing LP cells (areas of NLPHL) there were areas of atypical T-cells. 9 of these contained sheets of atypical T-cells surrounding primary and secondary follicles in a pattern mimicking the T-zone lymphoma of PTCL-NOS; the remaining 2 cases contained atypical T-cells presented as large clusters at the periphery of B-cell-rich nodules. The atypical T-cells showed no pan-T-cell antigen loss or aberrant T-cell antigen expression in any case, and PCR or Southern blot analysis showed no evidence of T-cell clonality in 6 cases tested. In comparision with control patients, NLPHL patients with atypical T-cells were more likely to develop recurrent NLPHL (71.4% vs. 13.6%, p=0.008) and to have a shorter time to relapse (p=0.04).

In CHL, together with genetic lesions affecting the neoplastic population, the malignant component is tightly regulated by interactions with the microenvironment. [156] Of particular interest is the presence of biased T-cell populations in HL cases, evidence for a dis-regulation of T cell immune function. In this sense, a considerable fraction of infiltrating CD4+ T cells are regulatory (Treg) cells which have been shown to display immunosuppressive activity on HL Th2 cells. The monocyte/macrophages prove to be a major determinant of prognostic outcome, the higher the content of CD68+ macrophages in diagnostic biopsy samples, the greater the risk of progression after primary treatment and relapse, following autologous stem cell transplantation. On the other hand, patients with limited-stage disease and without elevated numbers of CD68+ cell have a long-term disease-free survival of 100% using current treatment strategies.

Despite significant advances in the treatment of HL, considerable long term toxicity of conventional therapies requires the development of new non-genotoxic therapeutic strategies. The insight into the molecular pathogenesis of HL is likely to help in development of these new strategies. [189]

PATHOGENESIS OF HODGKIN'S LYMPHOMA

Whereas Kaplan and Smithers [131] hypothesized that Hodgkin disease might represent an autoimmune process, DeVita [190] called it a lymphocyte civil war. Kay, [191] in a scanning electron microscopic study of Hodgkin's tissue, found that T-cells cause cytolysis of R-S cells in a definite sequential manner and defined the pathogenesis of Hodgkin's disease on the basis of "a war between T-lymphocytes and transformed macrophages". According to him, [191] the various histopathological subtypes of HD and their prognosis depend upon the relative strength of both the forces, i.e., T-lymphocytes versus HR-S cells, and the outcome of the war, respectively. The R-S cell/lymphocyte interaction was further defined by Payne et al., [97, 192] who observed an antigen dependent lymphocyte/ macrophage contact and proposed the involvement of a unique receptor system for this interaction.

The pathogenesis of HL is still largely unresolved, but only over the last 15 years significant advances regarding its molecular pathogenesis has been achieved; [189] the reason behind this delay being the lack of a specific lineage profile in combination with the low number of malignant mononuclear Hodgkin- and multinucleated Reed-Stenberg-(HRS-) cells in the affected lymph nodes that prevented for a long time both the identification of its cell of origin and of genomic and molecular defects. The HRS cells harbor genetic lesions that contribute to or cause increase in the activity of transcription factors of the NF-kappaB and STAT families. [122] This aberrant activation of several signaling pathways (such as the NFkappaB pathway) is of key importance for HRS cell survival [121] because they protect HRS cells from apoptotic cell death. [189, 193] According to Schmitz et al., [122] HRS cells are found within a mixed reactive cellular infiltrate and interact with these non-malignant cells in a complex fashion that appears to be essential for HRS cell survival and proliferation; less is known about the pathogenesis of L&H cells in NLPHL, but an increase in the activity of receptor tyrosine kinase, NF-kappaB, and JAK/STAT has also been detected. NF-kappaB triggers proliferation and provides a molecular basis of cells' aberrant growth and cytokine gene expression. In HL pathogenesis associated with Epstein-Barr virus (EBV) infection, the activation of NF-kappaB is induced by viral latent protein 1 (LMP1); CD99 is down-regulated by LMP1 through NK-kappaB signaling pathway, which leads to the generation of cells with H-RS phenotypes related to the clinical and histologic characteristics of HL. [193]A biological link between 2 characteristic features of H-RS cells: CD30 overexpression and constitutive NF-kappaB activation has been observed; ligand-independent signaling by over expressed CD30 was shown to be a common mechanism that induced constitutive NF-kappaB activation in these cells, which suggest the self-growth-promoting potential of H-RS cells and redefine the biology of HL composed of H-RS cells and lymphocytes. [194]

With the above mentioned background information the molecular pathogenesis of Hodgkin's lymphoma can be explained as follows: There is compelling evidence that HRS cells are clonal B-cells that have lost their B-cell phenotype. [12] In other words, with the description of clonally rearranged immunoglobulin (Ig) genes with a high frequency of somatic mutations it has become clear that HRS cells are in most cases derived from germinal center (GC) or post GC B-cells, and despite their B-cell origin, HRS cells have, in most cases, lost the B-cell-specific gene expression program. [123] According to Yurchenko and Sidarenko, [195] due to reprogramming of gene expression, these lymphoma cells have lost the expression of most B-cell specific genes and acquired expression of multiple genes that are typical for other hematopoietic cells. According to Janz and Mathas, [123] the genomic alterations in HRS cells include activation of the transcription factor kappa B (NF-κB), activator protein 1 (AP-1), members of the STAT signaling pathway and deregulated NOTCH1 signaling; the NF-κB and AP1 transcription factors are thought to synergistically regulate not only genes involved in apoptosis protection and proliferation but also the abundant number of cytokines and chemokines produced by HRS cells. Furthermore, the AP1 and NOTCH1 signaling pathways have been shown to be involved in the loss of B-cell phenotype, characteristic of the HRS cells. Normally mature GC B-cells lacking functional B-cell receptors (BCR) complex would die by apoptosis, and therefore, the survival of HRS cells in the face of apoptotic triggers is considered central to CHL oncogenesis. The escape from apoptosis and transcriptional reprogramming of HRS cells are interlinked and appear central to the pathogenesis of Hodgkin lymphoma [12]: Epstein-Barr virus (EBV) is present in the HRS cells of a proportion of cases and express genes with plausible oncogenic function. It is likely that EBV plays a role in reprogramming and survival through dysregulation of several signaling networks and transcription factors, including nuclear factor (NF)-κB. Activation of NF-κB is a feature of all HRS cells and mutations affecting this pathway appear common in EBV-negative HL. The HRS cell furthers its own survival by attracting a supportive microenvironment of immune and stromal cells, and suppressing local immune responsiveness. The stromal background of HL include non-malignant T and B lymphocytes, plasma cells, histiocytes/macrophages, granulocytes, eosinophils, mast cells, interdigitating reticulum cells and fibroblast cells in collagen bands. [196] HRS cells can express and secrete a variety of cytokines, including IL-1, IL-2—IL-10, IL-13, IL-15, IL-21, ganulocyte-macrophage-colony-stimulating factor (GMCF), lymphotoxin-alpha (LF-α), transforming growth factor–beta (TGFβ), members of CCsubfamily of chemokines: CC chemokine ligand 5 (CCL5/RANTES), CCL17/TARC, CCL20, CCL22: and also a number of tumor necrosis factor (TNF) family cytokines (TNFα, BAFF, APRIL, RANKL, NGF). [196, 197] According to their functional role, cytokine in HL may be grouped in (1) attracting cells into microenvironment, (2) suppressing immune cells and (3) autocrine and/or paracrine regulators of HRS survival.

References

[1] Gruss HJ, Kadin ME. Pathophysiology of Hodgkin's disease: functional and molecular aspects. *Baillieres Clin Hematol* 1996; 9: 417-446.

[2] Hodgkin T. On some morbid appearances of the absorbent glands and spleen. *Med Chir Trans* 1832; 17:69-97.

[3] Wilks S. Cases of enlargement of the lymphatic glands and spleen (or Hodgkin's disease), with remarks. *Guy's Hosp Rep* 1865; 11:56-67.

[4] Sternberg C. Uber eine eigenartige unter dem Bilde der Pseudoleukamic verlaufende Tuberculose des lymphatischen Apparates. *Ztschr Heilk* 1898; 19:21-30.

[5] Reed DM. On the pathological changes in Hodgkin's disease, with special reference to its relation to tuberculosis. *Johns Hopkins Hospital Reports.* 1902; 10:133-136.

[6] Olu-Eddo AN, Omoti CE. Hodgkin lymphoma: Clinicopathologic features in Benin City, Nigeria and update on its biology and classification. *Nigerian J Clin Pract* 2011; 14:440-444.
[7] Cozen W, Katz J, Mack TM. Risk patterns of Hodgkin's disease in Los Angeles vary by cell type. *Cancer Epidemiol Biomarkers Prev* 1992; 1:261-268.
[8] Foss HD, Marafioti T, Stein H. Hodgkin lymphoma. Classification and pathogenesis. *Pathologe* 2000; 21: 113-123.
[9] Jaffe ES, Harris NL, Stein H, Vardiman JW, editors. World Health Organization classification of tumors. *Pathology and genetics of tumors of hematopoietic and lymphoid tissues.* Lyon: IARC Press; 2001.
[10] Lukes RJ, Craver LF, Hall TC, Rappaport H, Ruben P. Report of the nomenclature committee. *Cancer Res* 1966; 26:1311.
[11] Hartge P, Devesa SS, Fraumeni JF Jr. Hodgkin's and non-Hodgkin's lymphomas. *Cancer Surv* 1994; 19-20:423-453.
[12] Farrell K, Jarrett RF. The molecular pathogenesis of Hodgkin lymphoma. *Histopathology* 2011; 58:15-25.
[13] Landgren O, Caporaso NE. New aspects in descriptive, etiologic, and molecular epidemiology of Hodgkin's lymphoma. *Hematol Oncol Clin North Am.* 2007;21:825-840.
[14] Morton LM, Wang SS, Devesa SS, Hartge P, Weisenburger DD, Linet MS. Lymphoma incidence patterns by WHO subtype in the United States, 1992-2001. *Blood* 2006; 107:265-276.
[15] Eichenauer DA, Engert A, Dreyling M. Hodgkin's lymphoma: ESMO Clinical Practice Guidelines for diagnosis, treatment and follow-up. *Ann Oncol* 2011; 22 (S): vi55-58.
[16] Wu S-J, Chen C-Y, Su I-J, Tang J-L, Ko B-S, Huang S-Y, Yao M, Tsay W, Chen C-H, Tien H-F. Cliical characteristics and treatment response of Hodgkin's lymphoma in Taiwan. *J Formos Med Assos* 2008; 107: 4-12.
[17] Bastien H, Teisseyre A, Dusserre P, Michiels R, Cayot F, Lamy M, Cabanne F. Malignant lymphomas in Burgundy, France (1976--1977): a new approach using computerized pathological diagnoses. *Bull Cancer* 1979; 66:287-292.
[18] Radaszkiewicz T. Malignant and benign lymphomas: histologic classification and immunomorphologic studies. Results of 838 cases. *Wien Klin Wochenschr* 1980; 92:819-833.
[19] Kelényi G, Várbiró M. Malignant lymphoma reference centre—Hungary, 1978. *Virchows Arch A Pathol Anat Histol* 1980; 388:213-219.
[20] Shimizu M, Miura M, Kitahara M, Katayama I. Non-Hodgkin's lymphomas. Analysis of 109 Japanese cases with the use of LSGJ classification. *Am J Pathol* 1982; 106:30-39.
[21] Ho FC, Todd D, Loke SL, Ng RP, Khoo RK. Clinico-pathological features of malignant lymphomas in 294 Hong Kong Chinese patients, retrospective study covering eight-year period. *Int J Cancer* 1984; 34:143-148.
[22] Su IJ, Shih LY, Kadin ME, Dun P, Hsu SM. Pathologic and immunologic characterization of malignant lymphoma in Taiwan. With special reference to retrovirus-associated adult T-cell lymphoma/leukemia. *Am J Clin Pathol* 1985; 84:715-723.

[23] Calderon B, Villalon A, Augustion B, Jaier B, Zamuco J, Mori S Malignant lymphoma in Manila—a clinicopathologic study at the University of Philippines-Philippines General Hospital Medical Center. *Jpn J Clin Oncol* 1986; 16:21-27.

[24] Burla M, Egli F, Rhyner K. malignant lymphoma: a study of an outpatient cohort. *Schweiz Rundsch Med Prax* 1990; 79:101-110.

[25] Okpala IE, Akang EE, Okpala UJ. Lymphomas in University College Hospital, Ibadan, Nigeria. *Cancer* 1991; 68:1356-1360.

[26] Walter PR, Koltz F, Alfy-Gattas T, Minko-Mi-Etoua D, Nguembi-Mbina C. Malignant lymphomas in Gabon (equatorial Africa): a morphologic study of 72 cases. *Hum Pathol* 1991; 22:1040-1043.

[27] Ramani A, Kumar KA, Rao KK, Vidyasagar MS, Kundaje GN. Clinico-pathological profile of lymphomas in south India: a prospective rural hospital study of 103 cases. *J Assos Physicians India.* 1991; 39:322-325.

[28] Obafunwa JO, Akinsete I. Malignant lymphomas in Jos, Nigeria: a ten-year study. *Cent Afr J Med* 1992; 38:17-25.

[29] Ngendahayo P, Schmauz R. Pattern of malignant lymphoma in Rwanda. Bull Cancer 1992; 79:1087-1096.

[30] Ji X, Li W. Malignant lymphoma in Beijing. *J Environ Pathol Toxicol Oncol* 1992; 11:327-329.

[31] Yang K. A histopathologic and immunopathologic sudy of 209 malignant lymphoma cases from four regions of China: Suzhou, Nanjing, Qindao and Shenyang. *Zhonghua Zhong Liu Za Zhi* 1993; 15:86-90.

[32] Dasgupta A, Mukherjee C, Ghosh RN, Sengupta J. Malignant lymphoma—a 15-year study report. *J Indian Med Assos* 1993; 91:35-37.

[33] Cool CD, Bitter MA. The malignant lymphomas of Kenya: morphology, immunophenotype, and frequency of Epstein-Barr virus in 73 cases. *Hum Pathol* 1997; 28:1026-1033.

[34] Chai SP, Peh SC, Kim LH, Lim LY, Gudum HR. The pattern of lymphoma in east Malaysian patients as experienced in the University Hospital, Kuala Lumpur. *Malays J Pathol* 1999; 21:45-50.

[35] Chuang SS, Lin CN, Li C. Malignant lymphoma in southern Taiwan according to the revised European-American classification of lymphoid neoplasms. *Cancer* 2000; 89:1586-1592.

[36] Castella A, Joshi S, Raaschou T, Mason N. Pattern of malignant lymphoma in the United Arab Emirates—a histopathologic and immunologic study in 208 native patients. *Acta Oncol* 2001; 40:660-664.

[37] Getachew A. Malignant lymphoma in western Ethiopia. *East Afr Med J.* 2001; 78:402-404.

[38] Naresh KN, Agarwal B, Sangal BC, Basu DD, Kothari AS, Soman CS. Regional variation in the distribution of subtypes of lymphoid neoplasms in India. *Leuk Lymphoma.* 2002; 43:1939-1943.

[39] He S, Zhang JB, Zhang JG, Yang SY, Han F. The WHO (1997) classification of 370 cases of malignant lymphomas. *Zhonghua Xue Ye Xue Za Zhi* 2003; 24:519-522.

[40] Sukpanichnant S. Analysis of 1983 cases of malignant lymphoma in Thailand according to the World Health Organization classification. *Hum Pathol* 2004; 35:224-230.

[41] Haddadin WJ. Malignant lymphoma in Jordan: a retrospective analysis of 347 cases according to World Health Organization classification. *Ann Saudi Med* 2005; 25:398-403.

[42] Shivarov V, Dimitrov J, Guenova M. Lymphoid neoplasms in Bulgaria according to the WHO classification (2001). The experience of the National Center of Haematology. *Hematol J* 2005; 90:74-75.

[43] Wang JF, Wang YZ, Chen ZW, Taylor RC. Prevalence of lymphoma subtypes in Shaxi according to latest WHO classification. *Zhonghua Bing Li Xue Za Zhi* 2006; 35:218-223.

[44] Hashemi-Bahremani M, Parwaresch M-R, Tabrizchi H, Gupta RK, Raffii MR. Lymphomas in Iran. *Arch Iranian Med* 2007; 10:343-348.

[45] Jeong SY, Chang YH, Lee JK, Hong J, Hong SI, Lee SS. Incidence and histologic patterns of bone marrow involvement of malignant lymphoma based on the World Health Organization classification: a single institution study. *Korean J Lab Med* 2007; 27:383-387.

[46] Akhtar SS, Haque IU, Wafa SM, El-Saka H, Saroor AM, Nadrah HM. Malignant lymphoma in Al-Qassim, Saudi Arabia, reclassified according to the WHO classification. *Saudi Med* J 2009; 30:677-681.

[47] Yoon SO, Suh C, Lee DH, Chi H-S, Park CJ, Jang S-S, Shin H-R, Park B-H, Huh J. Distribution of lymphoid neoplasms in the Republic of Korea: Analysis of 5318 cases according to the World Health Organiztion classification. *Am J Hematol* 2010; 85:760-764.

[48] Mwakigonja AR, Kaaya EE, Heiden T, Wannhoff G, Castro J, PK F, Porwit A, Biberfed P. Tanzanian malignant lymphomas: WHO classification, presentation, ploidy, proliferation and HIV/EBV. *BMC Cancer* 2010; 10:344.

[49] Chen W-L, Tsai W-C, Chao T-Y, Sheu L-F, Chou J-M, Kao W-Y, Chen Y-C, Ho C-L. The clinicopathological analysis of 303 cases with malignant lymphoma classified according to the World Health Organization classification system in a single institute of Taiwan. *Ann Hematol* 2010; 89:553-562.

[50] Chakrabarti S, Sarkar S, Goswami BK, Mondal S, Roy A, Das S. Hodgkin's and non-Hodgkin's lymphoma in an rural medical institution: Comparative clinicopathologic analysis. *Asian Pac J Cancer Prev* 2010; 11:1605-1608.

[51] Jayasekara H, Karahalios A, Juneja S, Thursfield V, Farrugia H, English DR, Giles GG. Incidence and survival of lymphohematopoietic neoplasms according to the World Health Organization classification: a population-based study from the Victorian Cancer Registry in Australia. *Leuk Lymphoma* 2010; 51:456-468.

[52] Yago RT, Hughson MD, Sulayvani FK, Al-Allawi NA. Malignant lymphoma in northern Iraq: A retrospective analysis of 270 cases according to the World Health Organization classification. *Indian J Cancer* 2011; 48:446-451.

[53] Yang Q-P, Zhang W-Y, Yu J-B, Zhao S, Xu H, Wang W-Y, Bi C-F, Zou Z, Wang X-Q, Huang J, Dai L, Liu W-P. Subtype distribution of lymphomas in Southwest China: Analysis of 6,382 cases using WHO classification in a single institution. *Diagn Pathol* 2011; 6:77.

[54] Matteo E, Barón AV, Chabay P, Porta J, Dragosky M, Preciado MV. Comparision of Epstein-Barr virus presence in Hodgkin lymphoma in Pediatric versus adult Argentine patients. *Arch Pathol Lab Med* 2003; 127:1325-1329.

[55] Jackson Jr H, Parker Jr F. Hodgkin's disease. *II Pathology New Eng J Med* 1944; 231:35-44.

[56] Lukes RJ, Butler JJ. The pathology and nomenclature of Hodgkin's disease. *Cancer Res* 1966; 26:1063-1083.

[57] Harris NL, Jaffe ES, Stein H, Banks PM, Chan JK, Cleary ML, Delsol G, De Wolf-Peeters C, Falini B, Gatter KC, et al. A revised European-American classification of lymphoid neoplasms: a proposal from the international lymphoma study group. *Blood* 1994; 84:1361-1392.

[58] Swerdlow SH, Campo E, Harris NL, Jaffe ES, Pileri S, Stein H, Thiele J, Vardiman JW. *WHO Classification of Tumours of the Haematopoietic and Lymphoid Tissues.* Lyon, France: IARC Press; 2008 : 312-316.

[59] Das DK, Gupta SK, Datta BN, Sharma SC. Fine needle aspiration cytodiagnosis of Hodgkin's disease and its subtypes. I: Scope and limitations. *Acta Cytol* 1990; 34:329-336.

[60] Das DK, Gupta SK. Fine needle aspiration cytodiagnosis of Hodgkin's disease and its subtypes. II: Subtyping by differential cell counts. *Acta Cytol* 1990; 34:337-341.

[61] Fuggle WJ, Crocker J, Smith PJ. A quantitative study of eosinophil polymorphs in Hodgkin's disease. *J Clin Pathol* 1984; 37:267-271.

[62] Crocker J, Jones EL, Curran RC. A quantitative study of α-naphthyl acetate esterase-positive cells in Hodgkin's disease. *J Clin Pathol* 1982; 35:1301-1306.

[63] Kadin ME, Gladstein E, Dorfman RF. Clinicopathologic studies in 117 untreated patients subjected to laparotomy for staging of Hodgkin's disease. *Cancer* 1971; 27:1277-1294.

[64] Gough J. Hodgkin's disease. A correlation of histopathology with survival. *Int J Cancer* 1970; 5:273-281.

[65] Farrer-Brown G, Bennet MHarrison CV, Millet Y, Jellife AM. The pathological findings following laparotomy in Hodgkin's disease. *Br J Cancer* 1971; 25:449-457.

[66] Wright DH. Lymphoreticular neoplasms: In *Tumors of a tropical country. A survey of Uganda* (1964-68). AC Templeton Ed. RRCR 1973; 41:270.

[67] Mehrotra RML, Wahal KM, Kushwaha MRS, Bagchi M, SarkarB. Hodgkin's disease: A clinicopathological study of 300 cases. *Indian J Cancer* 1977; 14:249-255.

[68] Das DK. *Cytomorphological, cytochemical and immunological characterization of lymphomas.* Doctoral thesis. Postgraduate Institute of Medical Education and Research, Chandigarh, India. 1983.

[69] Petrella T, Michiels JF, Michiels R, Collin F, Nabholtz JM, Friedman S, Fargeot P. CD15 antigen in Hodgkin's disease. *Pathol Res Pract* 1989; 185:886-890.

[70] Liang R, Choi P, Todd D, Chan TK, Choy D, Ho F. Hodgkin's disease in Hong Kong Chinese. *Hematol Oncol* 1989; 7:395-403.

[71] Soriano Rosas J, Lazos Ochao M, Rojo Medina J, Manrique JJ, Herrera Verdugo D. Hodgkin's disease in the Hospital General de México, Study of 309 cases. *Sangre (Barc)* 1990; 35:447-450.

[72] Carde P. Hodgkin's disease-I: identification and classification. *Br Med J* 1992; 305:99-102.

[73] Bernhards J, Fischer R, Hübner K, Schwarze EW Georgil A. Histological classification of Hodgkin's lymphoma. Results from the reference pathology of the German Hodgkin Trial. *Ann Oncol* 1992; S4:31-33.

[74] Chang KL, Albújar PF, Chen Y-Y, Johnson RM, Weiss LM. High prevalence of Ebstein-barr virus in the Reed-Sternberg cells of Hodgkin's disease occurring in Peru. *Blood* 1993; 81:496-501.
[75] Medeiros LJ, Greiner TC. Hodgkin's disease. *Cancer* 1995; 75:357-369.
[76] Rana R, Chopra R, Masih K, Zachariah A, Prabhakar BR, Mahajan MK. Hodgkin's disease: a clinicopathologic study. *Indian J Pathol Microbiol* 1995; 38:245-249.
[77] De Souza CA, Vassallo J, Lorand-Metze I. Hogkin's disease in Brazil: a clinicopathologic study. *Haematologica* 1997; 82:127-128.
[78] Peh SC, Looi LM, Pallesen G. Epstein-Barr virus (EBV) and Hodgkin's disease in a multi-ethnic population in Malaysia. *Histopathology* 1997; 30:227-233.
[79] Liu SM, Chow KC, Chiu CF, Tzeng CH. Expression of Epstein-Barr virus in patients with Hodgkin's disease in Taiwan. *Cancer* 1998; 83:367-371.
[80] Monterroso V, Zhou Y, Koo S, Glackin C, Bujan W, Medeiros LJ. Hodgkin's disease in Costa Rica: a report of 40 cases analyzed for Epstein-Barr virus. *Am J Clin Pathol* 1998; 109:618-624.
[81] Mourad W, Alsohaibani MO, Saddik M, Bazerbashi S. Epstein-Barr virus expression in Hodgkin's disease: Correlation with histologic subtypes and T and B lymphocyte distribution. *Ann Saudi Med* 1998; 18:296-300.
[82] Enblad G, Sandvej K, Sundström C, Pallesen G, Glimelius B. Epstein-Barr virus distribution in Hodgkin's disease in an unselected Swedish population. *Acta Oncol* 1999; 38:425-429.
[83] Macák J, Habanec B, Fabián P. Detection of Epstein-Barr virus in Hodgkin's lymphoma (patients in the Czech Republic). *Neoplasma* 2000; 47:156-161.
[84] Glavina-Durdov M, Jakic-Razumovic J, Capkun V, Murray P. Epstein–Barr virus encoded latent membrane protein-1expression in Hodgkin's disease. *British Journal of Cancer,* 2001; 84:1227–1234.
[85] De Oliveira DE, Bacchi MM, Abreu ES, Niero-Melo L, Bacchi CE. Hodgkin disease in adult and juvenile groups from two different geographic regions in Brazil. *Am J Clin Pathol* 2002; 118:25-30.
[86] Krugmann J, Tzankov A, Gschwendtner A, Fischhofer M, Greil R, Fend F, Dirnhofer S. Longer failure-free survival interval of Epstein-Barr virus-associated classical Hodgkin's lymphoma: a single-institution study. *Mod Pathol* 2003; 16: 566-573.
[87] Almasri NM, Khalidi HS. Epstein-Barr virus expression in Hodgkin's disease in Jordan. *Saudi Med* J 2004; 25:770-775.
[88] Vassalo J, Pinto Paes F, Augusto Soares F, Menezes Y, Aldred V, de Cássia Braga Ribeiro K, Correa Alves A. Histological classification of 1,025 cases of Hodgkin's lymphoma from the state of São Paulo, Brazil. *Sao Paulo Med J* 2005; 123:134-136.
[89] Steidl C, Connors JM, Gascoyne RD. Molecular pathogenesis of Hodgkin's lymphoma: increasing evidence of the importance of the microenvironment. *J Clin Oncol* 2011; 29:1812-1826.
[90] Hoffman GT, Rottino A. Phase microscopy studies of Hodgkins disease lymph nodes in relation to histogenesis of Sternberg-Reed cell. *Blood* 1950; 5: 74-78.
[91] Seif GSF, Spriggs AI. Chromosome changes in Hodgkin's disease. *J Natl Cancer Inst.* 1967; 39: 557-570.
[92] Rappaport H. *Tumors of the hematopoietic system. Atlas of tumor pathology.* Section III. Fascicle 8. Armed Forces Institute of Pathology, Washington DC, 1966.

[93] Dorfman RF. Enzyme histochemistry of cells in Hodgkin's disease and allied disordes. *Nature* 1961; 190: 925-926.

[94] Order S, Hellman S. Pathogenesis of Hodgkin's disease. *Lancet* 1972; I: 571-572.

[95] Biniaminov M, Ramos B. Possible T-lymphocyte origin of Reed-Sternberg cells. *Lancet* 1974; I; 368.

[96] Herva E, Ryhanen P, Banco G, Jarvenppa K, Helin H, Alavaiko M. Acid alpha-naphthyl aetate esterase (ANAE) activity and DNA synthesis of lymph node cells in Hodgkin's disease. *Scand J Haematol* 1979; 23: 277- 284.

[97] Payne SV, Jones DB, Wright DH. Reed-Sternberg cells/lymphocyte interaction. *Lancet* 1977; II: 768-769.

[98] Leech J. *Immunoglobulin positive Reed-Sternberg cells in Hodgkin's disease.* 1973; II: 265-266.

[99] Taylor CR. An immunohistological study of follicular lymphoma, reticulum cell sarcoma and Hodgkin's disease. *Eur J Cancer* 1976; 12: 61- 75.

[100] Berneau D, Fildmann G, Vorhauer W. Hodgkin's disease. Ultrastructural localisation of intracytoplasmic immunoglobulins within malignant cells. *Br J Haematol* 1978; 40: 51-57.

[101] Papadimitrou CS, Stein H, Lennert K. The complexity of immunohistochemical staining pattern of Hodgkin and Sternberg-Reed cells: demonstration of immunoglobulin, albumin, alpha 1-antichymotrypsin and lysozyme. *Int J Cancer* 1978; 21: 531-541.

[102] Kadin ME, Stites DP, Levy R, Warnke R. Exogeneous immunoglobulin and the macrophage origin of Reed-Sternberg cells in Hodgkin's disease. *N Engl J Med* 1978; 299: 1208-1214.

[103] Kaplan HS, Gartner S. "Sternberg Reed" giant cells of Hodgkin's disease. Cultivation in vitro, heterotransplantation and characterization as neoplastic macrophages. *Int J Cancer* 1977; 19: 511-525.

[104] Long JC, Zamecnik PC, Aisenberg AC, Atkins L. Tissue culture studies in Hodgkin's disease. *J Exp Med* 1977; 145: 1484-1500.

[105] Kaplan HS. Hodgkin's disease: Unfolding concepts concerning its nature, management and prognosis. 1980; 45: 2439-2474.

[106] Poppema S, Elema JD, Haile MR. The significance of intracytoplasmic proteins in Reed-Sternberg cells. *Cancer* 1978; 42: 1973-1803.

[107] Maksem JA, Hassan MO, Carter JR. The ultrastrutural heterogeneity of the Reed-Sternberg cell and its resemblance to monocyte-macrophage differentiation in vivo. *Ultrastruct Pathol* 1983; 4:379-389.

[108] Diehl V, Burrichter H, Schaadt M, Kirchnner HH, Fonatsch C, Stein H, Gerdes J, Heit W, Ziegler A. Hodgkin's cell lines: characteristics and possible pathogenetic implications. *Hematol Oncol* 1983; 1:139-147.

[109] Drexler HG, Gignac SM, Hoffbrand AV, Minowada J. Formation of multinucleated cells in a Hodgkin's-disease-derived cell line. *Int J Cancer* 1989; 43:1983-1090.

[110] Marafioti T, Hummel M, Foss HD, Laumen H, Korbjuhn P, Anagnostopoulos I, Lammert H, Demel G, Theil J, Wirth T, Stein H. Hodgkin and Reed-Sternberg cells represent an expansion of a single clone originating from a germinal center B-cell with functional immunoglobulin gene rearrangements but defective immunoglobulin gene transcription. *Blood* 2000; 95: 1443-1450.

[111] Drexler HG. Recent results on the biology of Hodgkin and Reed-Sternberg cells. I. Biopsy material. *Leuk Lymphoma* 1992; 8: 283-313.
[112] Wachi E, Nakamura N, Abe M, Wasaka H. Hodgkin's disease with CD20 (B1) positive Reed-Sternberg cells—an immunohistochemical and immunoelectron microscopic study. *Fukushima J Med Sci* 1989; 35:69-77.
[113] Schmid C, Pan L, Diss T, Isaacson PG. Expression of B-cell antigens by Hodgkin's and Reed-Sternberg cells. *Am J Pathol* 1991; 139:701-707.
[114] Zukerberg LR, Collins AB, Ferry JA, Harris NL. Coexpression of 223. CD15 and CD20 by Reed-Sternberg cells in Hodgkin's disease. *Am J Pathol* 1991; 139: 475-483.
[115] Chang KC, Chang Y, Jones D, Su IJ. Aberrant expression of cyclin A correlates with morphogenesis of Reed-Sternberg cells in Hodgkin's lymphoma. *Am J Clin Pathol* 2009; 132: 50-59.
[116] Bai MC, Jiwa NM, Horstman A, Vos W, Kluin PH, Van der Valk P, Mulink H, Walboomers JM, Meijer CJ. Decreased expression of cellular markers in Epstein-Barr virus positive Hodgkin's disease. *J Pathol* 1994; 174: 49-55.
[117] Siebert JD, McClure SP, Banks PM, Gulley ML. Hodgkin's disease, mixed cellularity type, with B-cell immunophenotype. Report of a case and review of literature. *Arch Pathol Lab Med* 1995; 119: 474-479.
[118] Stein H, Hummel M. Cellular origin and clonality of classic Hodgkin's lymphoma: immunophenotypic and molecular studies. *Semin Hematol* 1999; 36: 233-241.
[119] Küppers R, Rajewsky K. The origin of Hodgkin and Reed/Sternberg cells in Hodgkin's disease. *Annu Rev Immunol* 1998; 16: 471-493.
[120] Küppers R. Identifying the precursors of Hodgkin and Reed-Sternberg cells in Hodgkin's disease: role of the germinal center B-cell lymphomagenesis. *J Acquir Immune Defic Syndr* 1999; 21 Suppl: S74-S79.
[121] Küppers R, Hansmann ML. The Hodgkin and Reed-Sternberg cell. *Int J Biochem Cell Biol* 2005; 37: 511-517.
[122] Schmitz R, Stanelle J, Hansmann ML, Küppers R. Pathogenesis of classical and lymphocyte-predominant Hodgkin lymphoma. *Annu Rev Pathol* 2009; 4: 151-174.
[123] Janz M, Mathas S. The pathogenesis of classical Hodgkin's lymphoma: What can we learn from analyses of genomic alterations in Hodgkin and Reed-Sternberg cells? *Hematologica* 2008; 93:1292-1295.
[124] Aisenberg AC, Wilkes BM. Lymph node T cells in Hodgkin's disease: analysis of suspensions with monoclonal antibody and resetting techniques. *Blood* 1982; 59:522-527.
[125] Facchetti F, De Wolf-Peeters C, van den Oord JJ, Desmet VJ. Plasmacytoid monocytes (so called plasmacytoid T cells) I Hodgkin's disease. *J Pathol* 1989; 158:57-65.
[126] Wise NB, Poston MA. Co-existence of brucella infection and Hodgkin's disease: clinical, bacteriologic and immunologic study. *JAMA* 1940; 155:1976-1984.
[127] Benda C. *Zur histology der pseudoleukamischen: Verhandl deut-pathology-Gessel.* 1904; 7:123-131.
[128] Warthin AS. Genetic neoplastic relationships of Hodgkin's disease, aleukemic and leukemic lymphoblastoma and mycosis fungoides. *Am Surg* 1931; 93:153-161.
[129] Gall EA, Mallory TB. Malignant lymphoma. A clinicopathologic survey of 618 cases. *Am J Pathol* 1942; 18:381-429.
[130] Chevalier P, Bernard J. *La Maladie de Hodgkin. Pans*, Messon.

[131] Kaplan HS, Smithers DW. Aut0immunity in man and homologous disease in mice in relation to the malignant lymphoma. *Lancet* 1959; 2:1-4.

[132] Peckham MJ. Quantitative cytology and cytochemistry of Hodgkin's tissue labelled in vivo with tritiated thymidine. *Br J Cancer* 1973; 28: 332-339.

[133] Schiffer LM. Proliferation of cells in Hodgkin's disease. *Natl Cancer Inst Monogr* 1973; 36: 191-194.

[134] Kadin ME, Ausberg AK. Long term cultures of Hodgkin's tissue: A morphologic and radioautographic study. *Lab Invest* 1973; 28:181-184.

[135] Whitelaw DM. Chromosome complement of lymph node cells in Hodgkin's disease. *Can Med Assos J.* 1969; 101: 74-81.

[136] Olinici CD. Cytogenetic observation in different cell lines in Hodgkin's disease. *Acta Cytol (Basel)* 1972; 48: 283-287.

[137] Harris NL, Jaffe ES, Diebold J, Flandrin G, Muller-Hermelink HK, Vardiman J. Lymmphoma classification—from controversy to consensus: The REA and WHO classification of lymphoid neoplasms. *Ann Oncol* 2000; 11 (Suppl 1):3-10.

[138] Lymphoma Study Group of Japanese Pathologists (No name listed). The World Health Organization classification of malignant lymphomas in Japan: Incidence of recently recognized entities. *Pathol Int* 2000; 50:696-702.

[139] Makar RR, Saji T, Junaid TA. Epsein-Barr virus expression in Hodgkin's lymphoma in Kuwait. *Pathol Oncol Res* 2003; 9:159-165.

[140] De Matteo E, Barón AV, Chabay P, Porta J, Dragosky M, Preciado MV. Comparision of Epstein-Barr virus presence in Hodgkin's lymphomain pediatric versus adult Argentine patients. *Arch Pathol Lab Med* 2003; 127:1325-1329.

[141] Zhang J-R, Raza AS, Greaves TS, Cobb CJ. Fine-needle aspiration diagnosis of Hodgkin lymphoma using current WHO classification-Re-evaluation of cases from 1999-2004 with new proposals. *Diagn Cytopathol* 2006; 34:397-402.

[142] Lee M-Y, Tan T-D, Feng A-C, Liu M-C. Clinicopathological analysis of 598 malignant lymphomas in Taiwan: Seven-year experience in a single institution. *A J Hematol* 2006; 81:568-575.

[143] Keresztes K, Miltenyi Z, Bessenyei B, Beck Z, Szollosi Z, Nemes Z, Olah E, Illes A. Association between the Epstein-Barr virus and Hodgkin's lymphoma in the North-Eastern part of HungaryL Effects on therapy and survival. *Acta Haematol* 2006; 116:101-107.

[144] Al-Salam S, John A, Daoud S, Chong SM, Castella A. Expression of Epstein-Barr virus n Hodgkin's lymphoma in a population of United Arab Emirates nationals. *Leuk Lymphoma* 2008; 49:169-1777.

[145] Hundall SD, Betancourt E, Barnhart E, Patel J. Comparative flow immunophenotypic features of the inflammatory infiltrates of Hodgkin lymphoma and lymphoid hyperplasia. *Cytometry Part B* (Clin Cytometry) 2008; 74B:1-8.

[146] Fong D, Steurer M, Greil R, Gunsilius E, Spizzo G, Gastl G, Tzankov A. Hodgkin lymphoma in Tyrol--a population-based study. *Ann Hematol* 2009; 88:449-456.

[147] Tzankov A, Matter MS, Dirnhofer S. Refined prognostic role of CD68-positive tumor macrophages in the context of the cellular micromileu of classical Hodgkin lymphoma. *Pathobiology* 2010; 77:301-308.

[148] Sohani AR, Jaffe ES, Harris NL, Ferry JA, Pittaluga S, Hasserjian RP. Nodular lymphocyte predominant Hodgkin lymphoma with atypical T cells: a morphologic variant mimicking peripheral T-cell lymphoma. *Am J Surg Pathol* 2011; 35:1666-1678.

[149] Anagnostopoulos I, Hansmann ML, Franssila K, Harris M, harris NL, Jaffe ES, Han T, van Krieken JM, Poppema S, Marafioti T, Franklin J, Sextro M, Diehl V, Stein H. European Task Force on Lymphoma project on lymphocyte predominance Hodgkin disease: histological and immunohistological analysis of submitted cases reveals 2 types of Hodgkin disease with a nodular pattern and abundant lymphocytes. *Blood.* 2000; 96: 1889- 1899.

[150] Mani H, Jaffe ES. Hodgkin lymphoma: An update on it biology with newer insights into classification. *Clin Lymphoma Myeloma* 2009; 9:206-216.

[151] Slack GW, Ferry JA, Haserjian RP, Sohani AR, Longtine JA, Harris NL, Zukerberg LR. Lymphocyte depleted Hodgkin lymphoma: an evaluation with immunophenotyping and genetic analysis. *Leuk Lymphoma* 2009; 50:937-943.

[152] Pinkus GS, Said JW. Hodgkin's disease, lymphocyte predominance type, nodular—a distinct entity? Unique staining profile for L&H variants of Reed-Sternberg cells defined by monoclonal antibodies to leukocyte common antigen, granulocyte-specific antigen, and B-cell-specific antigen. *Am J Pathol* 1985; 118:1-6.

[153] Pinkus GS, Said JW. Hodgkin's disease, lymphocyte predominance type, nodular—further evidence for a B cell derivation. L&H variant of Reed-Sternberg cells express L26, a pan B cell marker. *Am J Pathol* 1988; 133:211-217.

[154] Poppema S. The nature of the lymphocytes surrounding Reed-Sternberg cells in nodular lymphocyte predominance and other types of Hodgkin's disease. *Am J Pathol.* 1989; 135: 351- 357.

[155] Kame OW, Gelb AB, Shibuya RB, Warnke RA. Leu 7 (CD57) reactivity distinguishes nodular lymphocyte predominance Hodgkin's disease from nodular sclerosing Hodgkin's disease, T cell-rich B cell lymphoma and follicular lymphoma. *Am. J. Pathol.* 1993.;142: 541-546.

[156] Montes-Moreno S. Hodgkin's lymphoma: A tumor recognized by its microenvironment. *Adv Hematol* 2011; doi:10.1155/2011/142395.

[157] Marafioti T, Hummel M, Anagnostopoulos I, Foss HD, Falini B, Delsol G, Isaacson PG, Pileri S, Stein H. Origin of nodular lymphocyte-predominant Hodgkin's disease from a clonal expansion of highly mutated germinal-center B cells. *N Engl J Med.* 1997; 337:453-458.

[158] Braeuninger A, Küppers R, Strickler J, Wacker HH, Rajewsky K, Hansmann ML. Hodgkin and Reed-Sternberg cells in lymphocyte predominant Hodgkin disease represent clonal populations of germinal centre-derived tumor cells. *Proc Natl Acad Sci U S A* 1997; 94:9337-9342.

[159] Rüdiger T, Jaffe ES, Delsol G, de Wolf Peeters C, Gascovne ED, Georgii A, Harris NL, Kadin ME, ac Lennan KA, Poppema S, Stein H, Weiss LE, Müller-Hermelink HK. Workshop report on Hodgkin's lymphoma and related disease ('grey zone'lymphoma). *Ann Oncol* 1998; 9 (S):s31-s38.

[160] Das DK, Gupta SK, Pathak IC, Sharma SC, Datta BN. Burkitt-type lymphoma: diagnosis by fine needle aspiration cytology. Acta Cytol 1987; 31:1-7.

[161] Yazdi HM, Burns BF. Fine-needle aspiration biopsy of Ki-1-positive large-cell anaplastic lymphoma. *Acta Cytol* 1991; 35: 306- 310.

[162] Caraway NP. Strategies to diagnose lymphoproliferative disorders by fine-needle aspiration using ancillary studies. *Cancer (Cytopathol)* 2005; 105: 432- 442.

[163] Banks PM. The distinction of Hodgkin's disease from T-cell lymphoma. *Seminar Diagn Pathol.* 1992; 9: 279-283.

[164] Tani E, Jahansson B, Skoog L. T-cell-rich B-cell lymphoma: Fine-needle aspiration cytology and immunocytochemistry. *Diagn Cytopathol.* 1998; 18: 1-4.

[165] Frizzera G. The distinction of Hodgkin's disease from anaplastic large cell lymphoma. *Seminar Diagn Pathol* 1992; 9:291- 296.

[166] Woodruff RD. Reviewing histologic diagnosis of lymphoma: comparision of original and review diagnoses in 269 cases. *Arch Pathol Lab Med* 1981; 105:573-576.

[167] Liu Y, Zhuang H, Liao X, Luo D, Cai X. Immunophenotype and differential diagnosis of Hodgkin's lymphoma. *Zhonghua Xue Ye Xue Za Zhi* 2002; 23: 524-527.

[168] Harris NL. Hodgkin's disease: classification and differential diagnosis. *Mod Pathol* 1999; 12: 159-175.

[169] Elgin J, Phillips JG, Reddy VV, Gibbs PO, Listinsky CM. Hodgkin's and non-Hodgkin's lymphoma: spectrum of morphologic and immunophenotypic overlap. *Ann Diagn Pathol* 1999; 3: 263-275.

[170] Das DK, Francis IM, Sharma PN, Sathar SA, John B, George SS, Mallik MK, Sheikh ZA, Haji BE, Pathan SK, Madda JP, Mirza K, Ahmed MS, Junaid TA. Hodgkin's lymphoma: diagnostic difficulties in fine-needle aspiration cytology. *Diagn Cytopathol.* 2009; 37: 564-573.

[171] Franke S, Wlodarska I, Maes B, Vandenberghe P, Achten R, Hagemeijer A, De Wolf-Peeters C. Comparative genomic hybridization pattern distinguishes T-cell/histiocyte-rich B-cell lymphoma from nodular lymphocyte predominance Hodgkin's lymphoma. *Am J Pathol* 2002; 161:1861-1867.

[172] Mourad WA, Al Nazer M, Tulbah A. Cytomorphologic differentiation of Hodgkin's lymphoma and Ki-1+ anaplastic large cell lymphoma in fine needle aspirates. *Acta Cytol* 2003; 47: 744-748.

[173] Marafioti T, Mancini C, Ascani S, Sabattini E, Zinzani PL, Pozzobon M, Pulford K, Falini B, Jaffe ES, Müller-Hermelink HK, Mason DY, Pileri SA. Leukocyte-specific phosphoprotein-1 and PU.1: two useful markers for distinguishing T-cell-rich B-cell lymphoma from lymphocyte predominant Hodgkin's disease. *Haematologica.* 2004; 89: 957- 964.

[174] Kusuda M, Toriyama K, Kamidigo NO, Itakura H. A comparision of epidemiologic, histologic, and virologic studies on Hodgkin's disease in Western Kenya and Nagasaki, Japan. *Am J Trop Med Hyg* 1998; 59:801-807.

[175] Jarrett RF. Viruses and Hodgkin's lymphoma. *Ann Oncol* 2002; 13:23-29.

[176] Jarrett RF. Hodgkin's disease. *Baillieres Clin Haematol* 1992; 5:57-79.

[177] Huang X, Nolte I, Gao Z, Vos H, Hepkema B, Poppema S, van den Berg A, Diepstra A. Epidemiology of classical Hodgkin lymphoma and its association with Epstein Barr virus in Nothern China. *PLOS One* 2011;6: e21152 [Epub].

[178] Weinreb M, Day PJ, Niggli F, Powell JE, Raafat F, Hesseling PB, Sceneider JW, Hartley PS, Tzortzatou-Stathopoulou F, Khalek ER, Mangoud A, El-Safi ER, Madanat F, Al Sheyyab M, Mpofu C, Revesz T, Rafii R, Tiedemann K, Waters KD, Barrantes JC, Nyongo A, Riyat MS, Mann JR. The role of Epstein-Barr virus in Hodgkin's disease from different geographical areas. *Arch Dis Child* 1996; 74:27-31.

[179] Benharroch D, Shemer-Avni Y, Myint YY, Levy A, Mejirovsky E, Suprun I, Shendler Y, Prinsloo I, Arad S, Rager-Zisman B, Sacks M, Gopas J. Measles virus: evidence of an association with Hodgkin's disease. *Br J Cancer* 2004; 91:572-579.

[180] Wiggill TM, Mantina H, Willem P, Perner Y, Stevens WS. Changing pattern of lymphoma subgroups at a tertiary academic complex in a high-prevalence HIV setting: a South African perspective. *Acquir Immune Defic Syndr* 2011; 56:460-466.

[181] Diehl V, Stein H, Hummel M, Zollinger R, Connors JM. Hodgkin's lymphoma: biology and treatment strategies for primary, refractory and relapsed cases. *Hematology Am Soc Hematol Educ Program* 2003; 225-247.

[182] Allemani C, Sant M, De Angelis R, Marcos-Gragera R, Coebergh JM, and the EUROCARE Working Group. Hodgkin's disease survival in Europe and the US: Prognostic significance of morphologic groups. *Cancer* 2006; 107:352-360.

[183] von Wasielewski R, Mengel M, Fischer R, Hansmann ML, Hübner F, Franklin J, Tesch H, Paulus U, Werener M, Diehl V, Geogii A. Classical Hodgkin's disease. Clinical impact of the immunophenotype. *Am J Pathol* 1997; 151: 1123-1130.

[184] Smolewski P, Niewiadomska H, Los E, Robak T. Spontaneous apoptosis of Reed-Sternberg and Hodgkin cells; clinical and pathological implications in patients with Hodgkin's disease. *Int J Oncol* 2000; 17: 603-609.

[185] Oudejans JJ, Jiwa NM, Meijer CJ. Epstein-Barr virus in Hodgkin's disease: more than just an innocent bystander. *J Pathol* 1997; 181: 353-356.

[186] Keegan TH, Glaser SL, Clarke CA, Gulley ML, Craig FE, Digiuseppe JA, Dorfman RF, Mann RB, Ambinder RF. Epstein-Barr virus as a marker of survival after Hodgkin's lymphoma: a population-based study. *J Clin Oncol* 2005; 23: 7604-7613.

[187] von Wasielewski R, Seth S, Franklin J, Fischer R, Hübner K, Hansmann ML, Diehl V, Georgii A. Tissue eosinophilia correlates strongly with poor prognosis in nodular sclerosing Hodgkin's disease, allowing for known prognostic factors. *Blood* 2000; 95:1207-1213.

[188] Zaki MAA, Wada N, Iked J, Shibayaa H, Hashimoto K, Yamagami T, Tatsumi Y, Tsukaguchi M, Take H, Tsudo M, Morii E, Aozasa K. Prognostic implication of type of tumor-associated macrophages in Hodgkin lymphoma. *Virchows Arch* 2011; 459:361-366.

[189] Mathas S, Dörken B, Janz M. The molecular pathogenesis of classical Hodgkin lymphoma. *Dtsch Med Wochenschr* 2009; 134: 1944-1948.

[190] De Vita VT. Lymphocyte reactivity in Hodgkin's disease: lymphocyte civil war. *N Engl J Med* 1973; 289: 801-802.

[191] Kay MMB. Hodgkin's disease: A war between T-lymphocytes and transformed macrophages. *Monographs on lymphocytes, macrophages and cancer.* RRCR1976; 56:111-121.

[192] Payne SV, Nowell DG, Jones DG, Wright DH. The Reed-Sternberg cell lymphocyte interaction: Ultrastructure and characteristic of binding. *Am J Pathol* 1980; 100: 7-24.

[193] Lee IS, Kim SH, Song HG, Park SH. The molecular basis for the generation of Hodgkin and Reed-Sternberg cells in Hodgkin's lymphoma. *Int J Hematol* 2003; 77: 330-335.

[194] Horie R, Higashihara M, Watanabe T. Hodgkin's lymphoma and CD30 signal transduction. *Int J Hematol* 2003; 77: 37-47.

[195] Yurchenko M, Sidorenko SP. Hodgkin lymphoma: The role of cell surface receptors in regulation of tumor cell fate. *Exp Oncol* 2010; 32:214-223.

[196] Aldinucci D, Gloghini A, Pinto A, De Filippe R, Carbone A. The classical Hodgkin's lymphoma microenvironment and its role in promoting tumor growth and immune escape. *J Pathol* 2010; 221:248-263.
[197] Skinnider BF, Mak TW. The role of cytokines in classical Hodgkin lymphoma. *Blood* 2002; 99:4283-4297.

In: Hodgkin's and T-Cell Lymphoma
Editors: Warren K. Harvey and Randall M. Jacobs
ISBN 978-1-62257-478-0

Chapter 2

TREATING CUTANEOUS T-CELL LYMPHOMA: TOTAL SKIN ELECTRON BEAM THERAPY

Stefanos Diamantopoulos[1*], Kalliopi Platoni[1], Efstathios Efstathopoulos[1] and George Panayiotakis[2]
[1]Radiation Therapy Unit, 2nd Department of Radiology,
University General Hospital Attikon, Athens, Greece
[2]Medical Physics Department, Medical School,
University of Patras, Patras, Greece

ABSTRACT

Cutaneous T-cell Lymphoma is a relatively rare dermatological disease, with whole body symptomatology. The organ being mostly affected is the skin, without excluding internal organ involvement in progressed stages of the disease. For the cure of this type of lymphoma, several treatments have been employed. Fractionated irradiation of the whole skin surface, by high energy electrons, is one of the suggested therapeutic courses, either as exclusive or supplementary treatment. This method of external radiation therapy is commonly referred to in bibliography as Total Skin Electron Beam (TSEB) treatment. Every currently applied TSEB technique is based on a fundamental principle: the utilization of a homogeneous broad electron beam that can cover the patient in height and width. Due to their physical properties, high energy electrons (4-9 MeV) are appropriate for treating superficial lesions, while sufficiently wide fields can be generated by increasing the distance of the patient from the electron source (SSD > 3m). Such a beam can be produced by every commercially available linear accelerator, equipped with electron scattering foils. Nevertheless, the establishment of a total skin treatment protocol in a radiation therapy unit is a rather complex procedure. Unconventional patient positioning increases the number and frequency of quality checks. In addition, specially designed equipment is necessary for patient immobilization and support. Subsequently, only a limited number of health centers worldwide provide this kind of radiation therapy. Existing TSEB techniques are categorized depending on the manner of irradiation (standing, rotating-on-platform or reclined patient) and the number of required fields for

* E-mail address: diamantopstef@gmail.com

total skin coverage. Despite the variety of irradiation setups, over 80% of the clinics already providing TSEB have adopted a "six dual-field" arrangement. A critical safety aspect of TSEB is to minimize exposure of the patient to contaminating Bremsstrahlung radiation, derived from electrons interacting with parts of the linear accelerator's head. Therapeutic doses range between 20-40 cGy on skin, with the majority of centers prescribing an average of 36 cGy in a 9 week treatment scheme. In our institute, a "six dual-field" TSEB technique was developed, following international guidelines of radiation safety and dose prescription. A uniquely designed immobilization system was constructed by our clinic, equipped with a PMMA scatterer of proper dimensions. From the first clinical trial until now, all T-cell lymphoma patients being submitted into our treatment protocol, presented positive preliminary results, even up to full remission of the disease in certain cases. During the six decades of its existence, Total Skin Electron Beam irradiation has proven to be a reliable and effective treatment, for cure or palliation of cutaneous T-cell lymphoma, especially in early stages of the disease.

1. Introduction

Cutaneous T-cell lymphoma (CTCL) is a general title that comprehends a wide-ranging group of rare, chronic, and progressive dermatological cancers caused by malignant clones of T helper cells (T_H cells or $CD4^+T$ cells), which are produced by the thymus gland and infiltrate the skin layers. Although being malignancies of the self-same type of cells, the assorted clinical presentations of CTCL have been referred in the relevant medical bibliography over the years with several terms (such as mycosis fungoides (MF), Sézary syndrome (SS), lymphoma or leukemia cutis etc), conditional on the characteristics of the principal sub-clones of the malignant T-cells. The organ being predominantly affected is the skin in its entirety, without excluding the involvement of internal organs in progressed stages of the disease. For CTCL confrontation, many treatments have been administered to patient's skin. Currently available therapeutic options are corticosteroids, cytostatics, biologics, phototherapy, etc [1-3]. Total skin electron beam (TSEB) treatment is a radiation therapy process, dedicated to the management of skin malignancies with whole body symptomatology. This method is available to physicians since 1951, when Trump et al. [4], first utilized narrow rectangular electron beams of 2 MeV, produced by a modified Van der Graaff generator, to treat patients suffering from mycosis fungoides. Since then, a variety of modifications has been inserted to the fashion of irradiation, mainly after the establishment of isocentrically-mounted linear accelerators in medical practice. Nowadays, TSEB has been evolved into a successful and efficient treatment alternative, with many variants among radiation therapy departments around the world.

TSEB therapy takes advantage of the physical and geometrical features of high-energy electron beams for the creation of a large and homogenous clinical field at a distance of several meters from the source of emission, aiming at delivering the prescribed dose to the skin of the patient. High-energy electron rays (4-9 MeV) are the optimal choice of particles for this kind of treatment, principally due to their relatively short practical range (R_p), a physical property that ensures superficial energy deposition into tissue [5, 6]. Such beams can be produced by almost every modern clinical linear accelerator.

Published clinical results on TSEB efficacy against cutaneous malignancies, during the last six decades, have rendered this practice as a treatment of choice for T-cell lymphoma remediation, even if the prescription of the irradiation sessions aims merely at palliative care [1]. The total number of clinics that offer TSEB treatment modality worldwide is limited. The complexity of application procedure and clinical performance, as well as the low rate of CTCL appearance in population, make the provision of a TSEB technique in every radiation therapy unit rather impractical [6]. Linear accelerator calibration and quality assurance (QA) programs for TSEB are different in many ways from the respective protocols performed for conventional electron radiation therapies. A complete new calibration sequence should be followed, depending on the specific features of each individual TSEB technique, while rigid and frequently executed QA checks should put the initially chosen parameters under test [6].

2. The Basics of TSEB Implementation

The installation of a total skin treatment protocol in a radiation therapy unit is a considerably complex procedure. Due to the by default unconventionally designed irradiation setup, additional devices are essential, (except to the already existing equipment in every radiation therapy department), not only for clinical performance of the treatment, but also for the installation measurements and the routine quality assurance program.

The suitable electron beam quality (4 to 9 MeV) can be produced by every commercially available medical linear accelerator, equipped with electron scattering foils (Figure 1). Nevertheless, treatment layout differs completely from commonly performed electron radiation therapies. As prescription target volume (PTV) is the entire skin surface (and the adjacent skin layers), the ultimate aim of TSEB treatment is to irradiate uniformly, with the prescribed dose, the skin to the desired depth, with the least (as low as reasonably achievable) concomitant and hazardous X-ray background. Hence, many modifications are introduced in irradiation geometry, linear accelerator's operational parameters, and patient positioning [6-8].

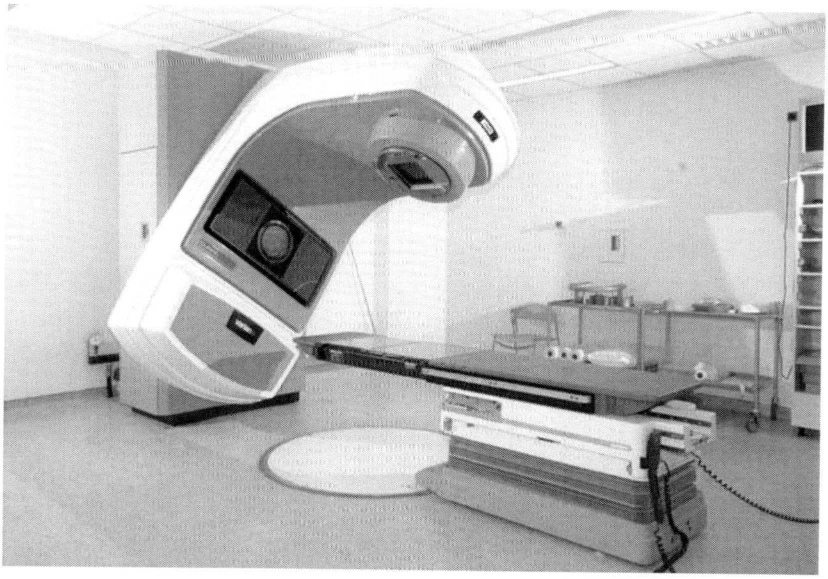

Figure 1. A typical medical linear accelerator system in a radiation therapy treatment room.

2.1. Clinical Field Properties

2.1.1. Energy of Electrons

The desired energy for TSEB treatment (most probable energy-E_p) should be 3 to 5 MeV at the plane of treatment. With this electron energy value, a penetration depth range (R_{50}) of 15 mm could be achieved. The majority of skin lesions (depending on the stage of the disease) are likely to be included within this range.

The rough estimation of electron energy loss of 2 MeV/(g/cm^2) undervalue the required energy for the desired depth of penetration, and should not be utilized for calculations, as numerous electrons did not cross the threshold of the skin surface vertically [6].

2.1.2. Dimensions of Clinical Field

Field size in TSEB treatment mode should be large enough in order to ensure whole body coverage. Therefore, suggested sizes of a clinical TSEB electron field are equal to or larger than 200 cm in height and 80 cm in width, at the treatment plane.

This implies that, in order to achieve an effective rectangular electron cross-sectional area of such length and breadth, collimator jaws should be widely open during irradiation to the maximum attainable dimensions. Some linear accelerators are equipped with special trays, dedicated for collimator adjusting to the appropriate aperture (34 x 34 cm^2 or 36 x 36 cm^2 projections at the isocenter). The dimensions of such fields do not permit the use of electron applicators, as required in typical electron therapies. As a result, the lack of field modulation entails irregular shaped and energy-dependent dose profiles [6].

2.1.3. Flatness of Clinical Field

A TSEB technique is considered clinical acceptable if an average ±5% variation of dose at depth of z_{max} in a phantom on the central ray for at least 80% of the nominal field area has been achieved. This directive could also be analyzed to vertical and horizontal flatness limits of ±8% and ±4% respectively, at the same field cross-section. The doubled tolerance limit value at vertical uniformity, in comparison to the horizontal dimension homogeneity limit, is attributed to the fact that in most TSEB techniques, more than one partial electron fields are combined to reach the longitudinal field dimension of 200 cm [6, 7].

2.2. Treatment Room Requirements

2.2.1. Source Skin Distance-SSD

The maximum achievable field dimensions, in every linear accelerator, are confined to a projection of 40 x 40 cm^2 at the mechanical isocenter plane. **As a consequence,** a single electron field is incapable of covering the proportions of an average-sized patient who is placed at a typical source-skin distance (SSD) of approximately 100 cm. Hence, TSEB is performed by utilizing an off-couch patient positioning, exploiting the geometrical properties in space of the electron beam. Nominal source-skin distance in every TSEB technique ranges between 2 to 7 meters [6].

Additionally, extended SSD offers the advantage of energy degrading of the clinical beam through the intermediate volume of air. Thus, shallow penetration of electrons into tissue is accomplished. Radiation therapy clinics, that intend to initiate a total skin treatment protocol, should meet these requirements of treatment room dimensions. In case of inadequacy of spatial comfort, a compromise on SSD and the number of component fields, which add up to the properly sized clinical TSEB field, should be reached. In general, the number of partial fields increases with the decreasing of SSD.

2.2.2. Room Ventilation

Sufficient air circulation is a basic room prerequisite. As produced electrons interact with air particles, an excessive amount of toxic ozone (O_3) is produced and released into the treatment room atmosphere, which should be ventilated adequately [6].

2.2.3. Room Surveillance

Room monitoring is imperative during beam-on time. Especially for techniques that the patient (in most cases, in his late adulthood) is standing up for prolonged periods, with his eyes shielded, taking inconvenient positions and, possibly, having lost his orientation, there is always the probability of losing balance and dropping off or even fainting [6].

2.2.4. Room Radiation Shielding

Normally, there is no need for additional shielding designs for the treatment room, as the existing one for therapeutic photon energies (at least 6 MV) suffices for the majority of TSEB techniques. Nevertheless, a verification measurement should be performed to confirm adequate radiation protection from TSEB practice [6].

2.3. Patient Positioning and Supporting Systems

For precision and repeatability in the daily positioning of the patient, a special immobilization and supporting device is compulsory. This apparatus should be equipped with grips, straps, belts, rotatable bars and any other kind of necessary auxiliary accessories, in order to provide stability to the patient and minimize the possibility of inadvertent movements during treatment, notably for TSEB techniques that require a "standing" patient treatment posture (see §4.1.–§4.2.).

These devices could be portable or strictly attached to the floor, the wall, or even the ceiling of the treatment room. Depending on the TSEB technique, they also could be rotated by platforms or equipped to motor driven couches. If the system is portable, then its correct placement at every session is achieved by guiding lines on the floor and marks in relation to treatment room lasers. On the other hand, the precise positioning of the patient is performed according to specially designed templates.

In most cases, the very same immobilization system serves as a framework for large panels made of tissue equivalent materials (PMMA, Lexan, Lucite etc), placed proximal and parallel to treatment plane, which function as filters for further energy reduction and scattering of the electron beam.

Furthermore, the system is able to bear the dosimetric equipment for QA performance, by attaching on it removable parts (shelves, plywood panels with coordinate systems, etc). Such devices can be commercially provided or custom-designed and construct, according to the special needs of each clinic [6] (Figure 2).

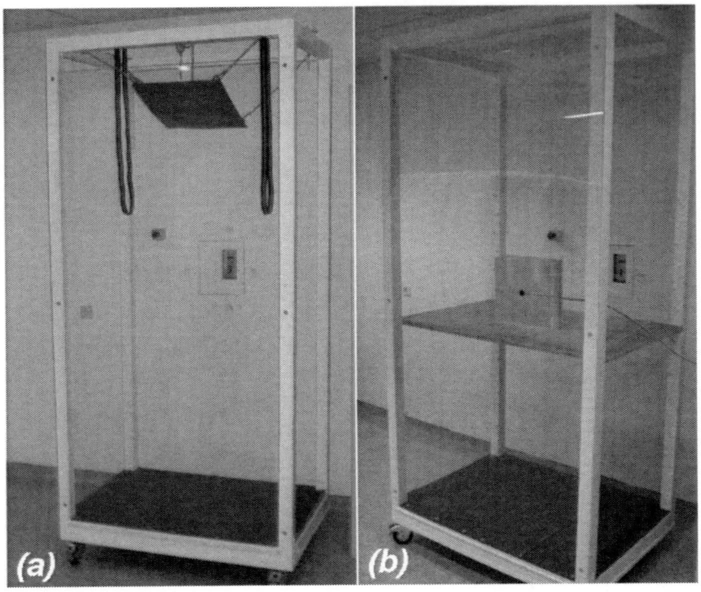

Figure 2. Originally designed and constructed immobilization system at the Radiation Therapy Department of University General Hospital "Attikon", Athens, Greece, dedicated for patients undergoing TSEB treatment [11] (a) Clinical use arrangement (b) QA performance arrangement; equipped with a removable self for measurement conducting.

2.4. Lead Shielding Equipment

The organs of increased radiosensitivity (such as eyes, finger and toe nails, genitals, etc) should be protected during beam-on time. Therefore, lead shielding of appropriate thickness has to be calculated and designed for these regions according to the dose prescription of radiation oncologists and the technique of treatment. The construction of shielding accessories is often complicated, as they are patient-tailored and their shape should molded to fit specifically to curvy and irregularly formed areas of the body (Figure 3).

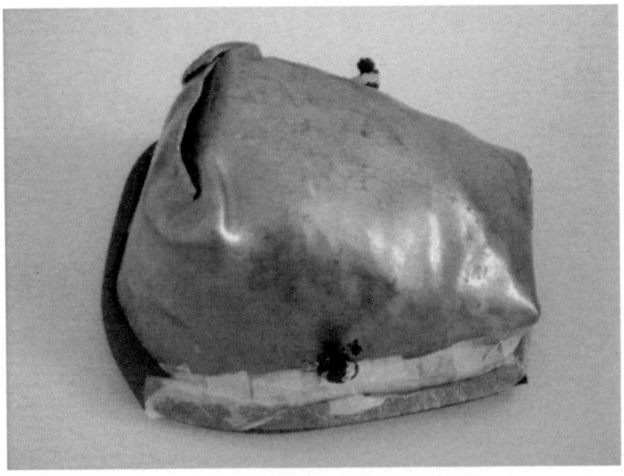

Figure 3. Handcrafted helmet, made by a lead sheet of 0.4 cm thickness, for scalp radiation protection during TSEB treatment.

In case of any change in the original technique setup, their thickness should be re-calculated. Especially for eye lens protection, in case of disease involvement of the eyelids, where an external shield would exclude them from treatment, lead cups should be applied internally, in contact to the lens.

The use of such a shield probably would raise the dose in the inner surface of the lids by a factor of 1.5 from backscattered particles on the high-Z lead; however, the benefit from eye lens protection is far more important. This equipment is commercially available or it can be prepared. Internal eye shields should always be escorted by auxiliary equipment, such as anesthetic eye drops and lubricants for their easy placement on the eye lens, and sterile dilutions for their storage and cleaning before and after use [6].

2.5. Quality Assurance Requisites

2.5.1. Instrumentation and Phantoms

For TSEB implementation and periodic performance of quality assurance (QA) tests, no need for sophisticated measurement equipment exists. Nevertheless, the off-couch setup necessitates the design of a series of application experiments and a QA program, based on international quality assurance protocols, dedicated to TSEB procedure exclusively and carefully adapted to the specific characteristics of each technique. Parallel-plate ionization chambers connected to concurrently calibrated electrometers are the proper dosimetric systems for electron beam monitoring (absolute and relative dosimetry) [5].

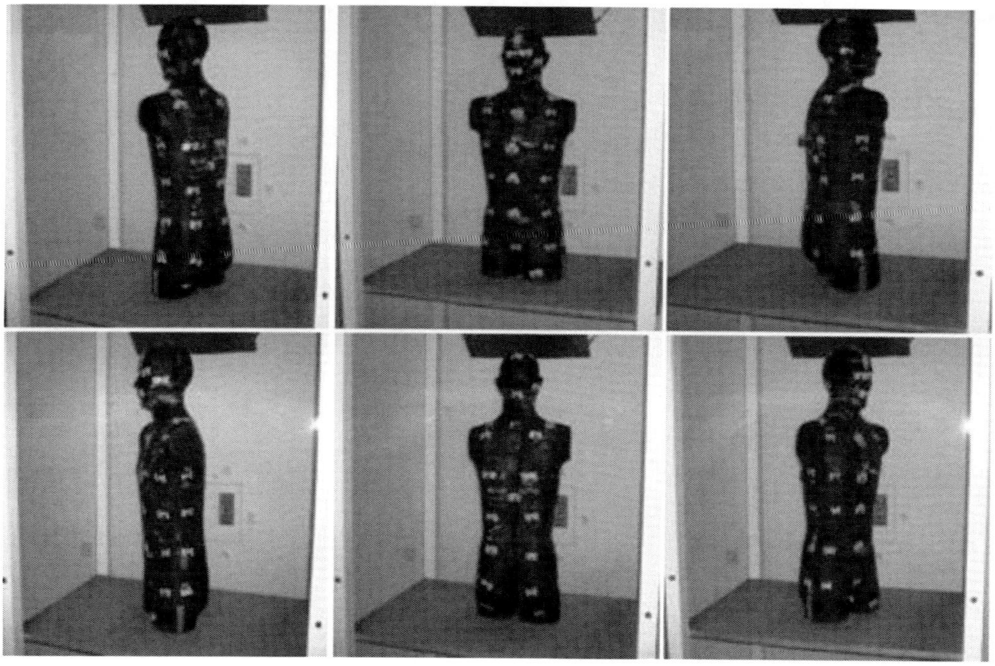

Figure 4. Utilization of an anthropomorphic phantom (Rando-Alderson phantom-male) for physical determination of dose distribution. Phantom positioning simulates the placement of the patient in actual clinical conditions. Dose uniformity measurements are achieved by TLD chips, distributed evenly on phantom's surface.

In addition, TLD or radiochromic film dosimeters, (calibrated at the TSEB beam quality with a parallel-plate electron ionization chamber) are necessary during TSEB installation and further quality assurance dosimetry. Water phantoms, solid-state polystyrene phantoms of flat or cylindrical shape and of human morphology (anthropomorphic) are necessary for both of the above-mentioned procedures [6, 7] (Figure 4).

2.5.2. Cable Effect

During every measurement process, incident electrons, on the part of the connection cable that is exposed to the clinical field, can alter the electrical signal of the ionization chamber (and, thus, the reading on the electrometer). This effect is universally referred to as the "cable effect" and it is present at electron field measurements.

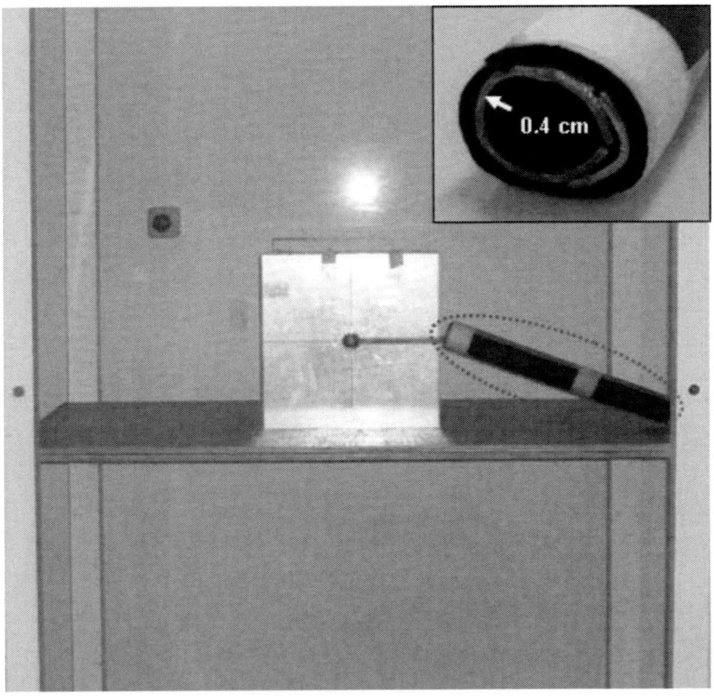

Figure 5. Experimental setup for the acquisition of the percentage depth dose (PDD) curve and the determination of the absorbed dose in various depths into tissue. The cable that connects the ionization chamber to the electrometer is shielded by a lead pipe (0.4 cm thick and 100 cm in length) in order to avoid measurement alteration caused by the "cable effect".

The magnitude and sign of charge values deviations depends on the polarity applied to the electrometer. For, e.g., measurements occurred with a parallel-plate ionization chamber of an electron beam with nominal energy of 6 MeV at an SSD of 380 cm, degraded by an acrylic sheet of 0.5 cm thickness, the falsification of charge data is -1.9% and +1.5% for positive (+150 V) and negative (-150 V) polarity respectively.

To avoid this phenomenon and for proper acquisition of the dose-related charge values, lead shielding around the part of equipment cables that is contained in the electron field during measurements, is essential [9-11] (Figure 5). The thickness of lead should be determined experimentally.

2.5.3. "In Vivo" Dosimetry

At any rate, an "in vivo" dosimetry practice should be developed (TLDs, films, diodes) for daily verification of the prescribed therapy, as no treatment planning system (TPS) is involved in the dose delivery procedure. The recorded results by this process, would reveal inhomogeneities in dose distribution, and, later, would guide the prescription of supplementary irradiation courses (see §5.3).

"In vivo" measurements of the dose should be preferably performed by radiochromic film dosimetry, as thereby, two-dimensional dose monitoring is achieved [12, 13] without interfering substantially to dose uniformity. Nevertheless, physicists should be aware that they are likely to absorb a minor percentage of the delivered dose, at the expense of the skin area underneath them. A simple and effective solution to this problem is to reduce film surface area for TSEB dosimetry and to slightly change their original position at each session, in order to eliminate local dose delivery complications. On the other hand, when radiochromic dosimetry equipment is not available, the utilization of TL dosimeters is a reliable method for "in vivo" dose recording. Calibration conditions of the "in vivo" dosimeters should simulate as much as possible the clinical setting for accurate and valid measurements. It is also recommended to use the same equipment (films or TLD chips) for "in vivo" measurements and for TSEB dosimetry.

3. Physical Parameters

The application of a "total skin electron beam" treatment mode at a health center requires three basic stages of calibration measurements and assessment of the obtained results. Physical determination of the large clinical electron field is the primary procedure, on which any other parameter should be adjusted accordingly.

Each and every geometric characteristic is analyzed and decisions on the final arrangement of equipment in the treatment room are taken. This step includes the choice of a particular TSEB technique, that will be applied, and the precise specification of nominal source-skin distance (SSD).

In addition, the exact dimensions of the stationary field at treatment plane are calculated along with beam energy, percentage depth dose, absorbed dose, dose profile, dose rate, and permissible levels of X-ray background radiation. Consequently, the cumulative dose and dose distribution derived from the total number of the contributing fields is evaluated. For this stage, tissue-mimicking phantoms are employed in conjunction with the available dosimetric equipment. Additionally, the time of dose delivery is estimated and the fraction of Monitor Units to dose units is defined.

The determination of clinical performance and dose prescription parameters are the third and final step of a TSEB installation process. The amount of the prescribed dose, dose fractionation and treatment intervals, boost fields for underdosed areas, shielding design, and quantification of integral Bremsstrahlung radiation [10] are some of the critical aspects that physicians and medical physicists should demarcate precisely for a safe and at the same time, effective radiation therapy.

4. CATEGORIZATION OF TSEB TECHNIQUES

Total skin electron beam therapy can be performed variously as long as the concept of the broad stationary electron field is applied. The existing diversity in TSEB treatment protocols and techniques has been developed over the years, to overcome technical restrictions, to exploit technological advance, and to serve the specialized features of each radiotherapy clinic. The triad of available space in each treatment room [14], routine session schedule [15-17], and patient comfort [18] encompasses the basic aspects that affect the choice of certain TSEB parameters during implementation. An apparent classification of TSEB techniques is based on patient placement in front of the linear accelerator. Thus, three main subcategories of TSEB can be distinguished: Standing, rotating, and reclined patient techniques.

4.1. Standing Patient Techniques

4.1.1. Single-Scattered Horizontal Beam

A large and homogenous field is produced by taking advantage of the geometrical features of electron rays. The patient is positioned at SSD of 7 m away from linear accelerator's head [6]. Energy modulation of the beam is achieved by the employment of energy degraders [19]. The basic materials that are utilized for their manufacture are acrylic, aluminum or titanium, either separately or in combination for better beam flattening. The main disadvantage of this technique is the necessity of a large treatment room.

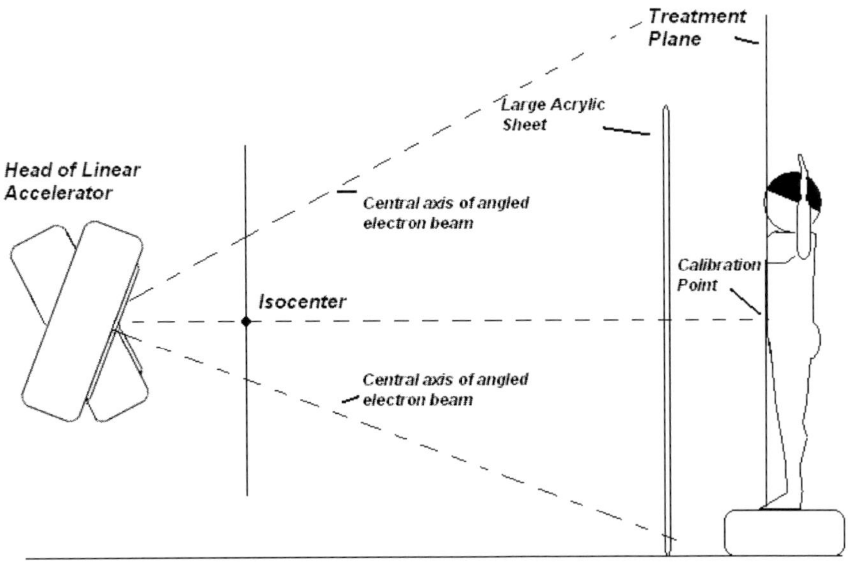

Figure 6. The typical clinical setup for multiple dual-field techniques.

4.1.2. Multiple Dual-Field Techniques

These techniques have been developed to eliminate the "large treatment room" limitation. A pair of angled electron beams composes a larger electron field. As a result, SSD is reduced to 3-4 meters. The relative angle is achieved by partial rotation of the gantry above and below of the horizontal direction, by averaging 20° degrees (Figure 6 and Figure 7). Patient is irradiated gradually by the composed stationary electron field at four (cross-pattern irradiation), six or eight (star-pattern irradiation) positions in front of the beam.

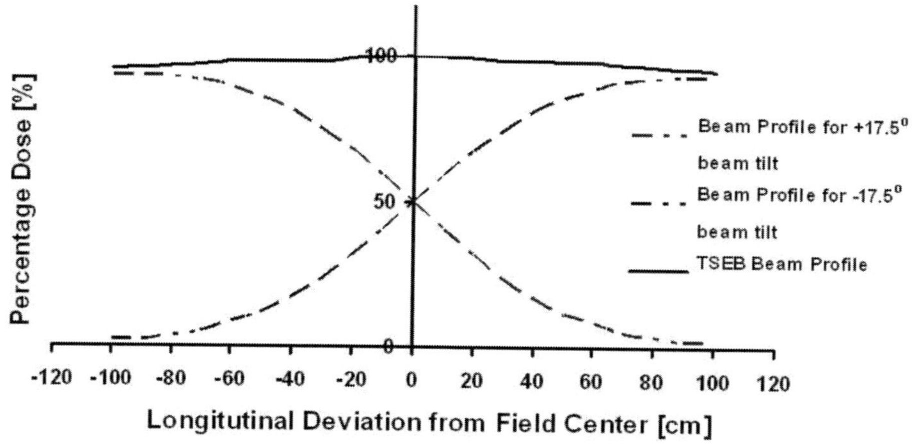

Figure 7. Composition of the clinical TSEB field dose profile at SSD = 380 cm by the summation of two angled electron beams at treatment plane [11].

At every position, there is a standard posture of patient's body, in order to expose to the treating beam the greatest portion of the malignant regions of the skin, minimizing the "self-shielding" effect. As a rule, dose uniformity improves with the increase of the total number of stances, at the cost of time for treatment carryied out.

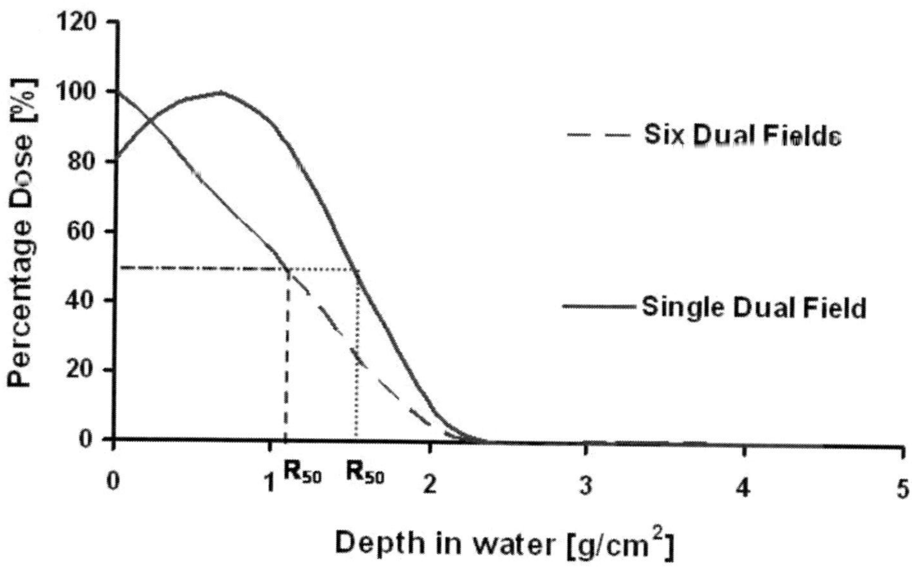

Figure 8. Percentage Depth Dose (PDD) curves derived from a single dual electron field and a complete six dual electron field irradiation. For the latter, superficial deposition of maximum electron energy is achieved. The difference in electron penetration into tissue is depicted by the difference between the two respective R_{50} depths [11].

The composite electron field is modulated by tissue-equivalent energy degraders, which are also able to scatter electrons for even better dose distribution. In addition, the multiple-field concept leads to shifting the depth of maximum dose deposition into tissue to shallower depths in comparison to a single field irradiation setup (Figure 8). This particular field arrangement provides a benefit in reducing contamination from Bremsstrahlung radiation as well. As this phenomenon is directional, and the greater proportion of produced X-rays is concentrated around the central axis of the electron beam, the applied angulations guide the majority of harmful photons outwards the trunk of the patient [6].

4.1.2.1. Six dual-field technique

The most common variation of this subgroup is the "six dual-field" or the "Stanford" technique. This routine is the best feasible combination of homogeneous dose distribution on skin with practical treatment time. The patient takes, in total, six positions of treatment, deviating from each other with 60° degrees angular intervals. A full irradiation cycle is completed in two days (some clinicians have adopted a three-day cycle), with patient taking three out of six positions at every session (Figure 9). Developed in the late 1960s by Stanford University, this technique was further modified in 1973 to allow the utilization of electron beams of higher energies.

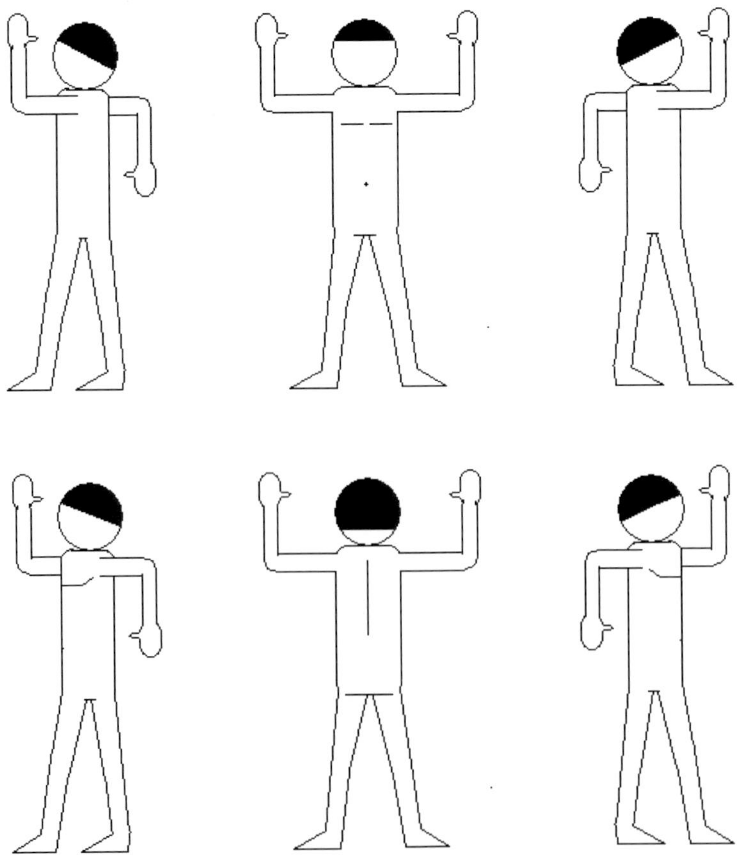

Figure 9. Standard treatment postures of the body of the patient in front of the clinical electron field for the six dual-field technique.

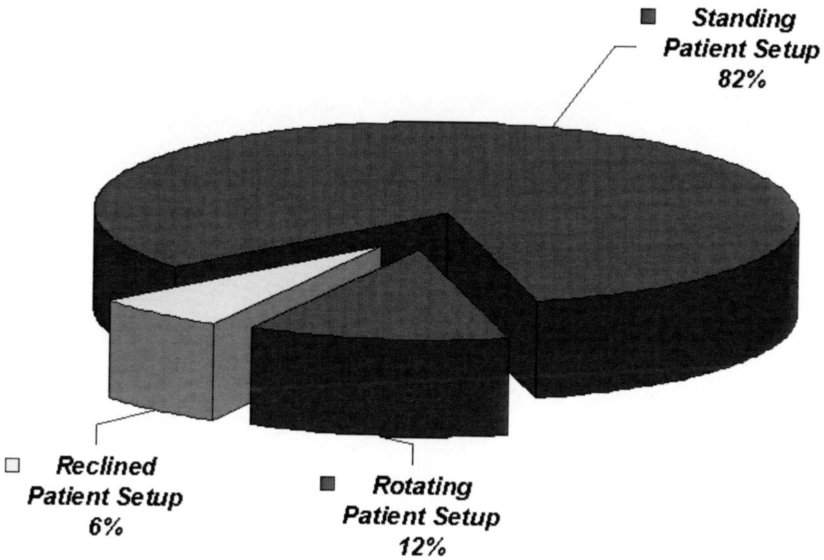

Figure 10. Worldwide percentage distribution of TSEB techniques depending on patient positioning during treatment.

At the present time, the "six dual-field" technique has evolved into the most widespread TSEB field arrangement (especially since the early 1990's [10, 20-39]), which, in some cases, have even replaced formerly established techniques [1, 6, 9, 12, 16-19, 34, 38-70].

This propensity is justified as the restrictive factor of small rooms is eradicated [31, 40], without compromising the dosimetric quality of treatment service [55]. The percentage of TSEB providing radiotherapy clinics that currently apply this irradiation technique worldwide exceeds 80%, according to bibliography (Figure 10).

4.2. Rotating Patient Techniques

The main idea of these TSEB techniques is to achieve the delivery of the prescribed dose to the entire skin surface by setting the patients on rotating platforms of stable angular speed. The electron beam is on during a full rotation of the patient. The large electron field is created by single- or dual-fields on the corresponding SSD (Figure 11).

Energy degraders and beam filters-scatterers properly shape the dose profile. Additional assisting equipment is necessary to provide support to the patient during rotation. The indisputable benefit gained by rotational TSEB is the achievement of relatively shorter treatment time in comparison to other currently applied techniques [15]. In addition, field junctioning related problems are removed, when the stability of angular speed of the rotating platform is guaranteed.

Nevertheless, "self-shielding" phenomena, mainly from the limps, are more frequent, due to the body posture of the patient during rotation process. The employment of rotational techniques worldwide reaches the percentage of 12% (Figure 10).

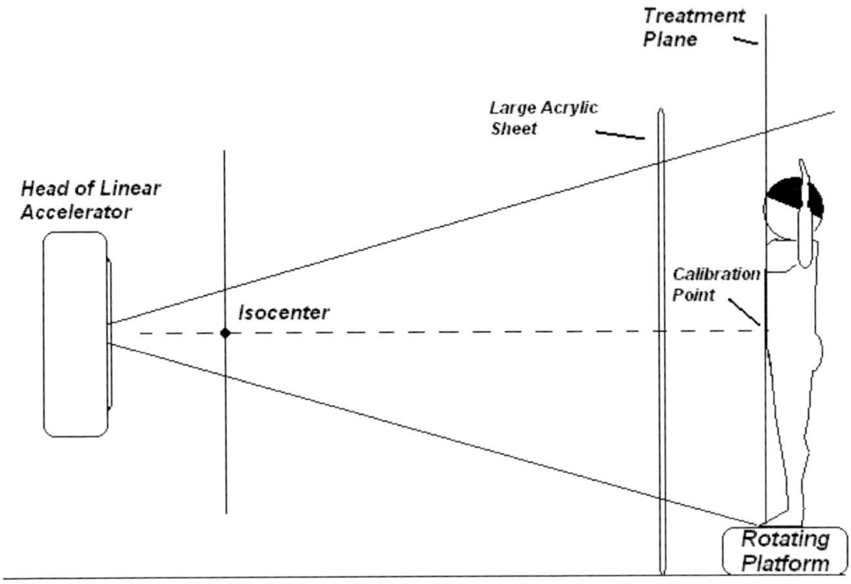

Figure 11. Typical clinical setup of rotating-patient techniques.

4.3. Reclined Patient Techniques

As their name indicates, at these particular irradiation methods, the patient is at a reclined position during beam-on time. These techniques constitute only a small percentage of all utilized TSEB modes. Although their use is not widespread, they provide a clear advantage on patient comfort and repeatability of the treatment setup. Reclined patient techniques can be further classified into the following modifications.

4.3.1. Translational Techniques

This specific TSEB treatment setup was originally employed in 1953 by Trump et al [71] for patients moving through narrow electron beams. Nowadays, the patient is lying on a couch on the floor that is driven mechanically through an electron field of proper energy, produced by the linear accelerator. As the SSD is restricted to head-floor distance, the "scanning" of body through motion accomplishes the full coverage of the anterior and posterior side of the skin [6, 42] (Figure 12).

Another TSEB type that is based on a similar setup is Christie Hospital technique, developed in Manchester, UK. Placed at the maximum possible SSD (150 cm) on the couch of linear accelerator, the patient slides perpendicular to the axis of the beam [38].

4.3.2. Lying-On Techniques

The patient is set on a stretcher on the floor and is irradiated utilizing a field coupling technique, based on multiple fields' physical principles. The large electron field is modified by a PMMA sheet, which is sustained over the patient by a properly designed supporting system. Oblique irradiation is achieved by an angulated position of the gantry and placement of the acrylic sheet, in order to be perpendicular to electron beam axis [18].

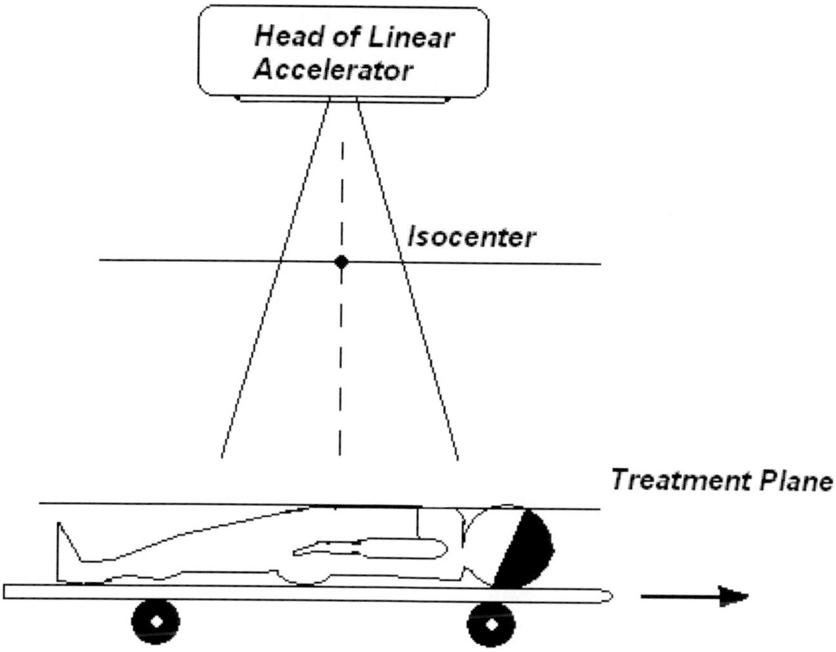

Figure 12. Typical clinical setup of translational techniques.

A slightly different technique that involves a reclined patient and stationary electron fields is a modification of the previously described Christie Hospital technique, which is applied at the Northern Israel Oncology Center.

The patient is lying on a couch at a source-skin distance of 150 cm. The matching of four to five pairs (depending on the height of the patient) of angled electron beams leads to the complete coverage of the patient's surface [38]. The main drawbacks of this technique are the enlargement of dose delivery time and the insertion of greater uncertainty in field junction areas when compared to other TSEB techniques. Nevertheless, the on-couch setup solves any kind of space, complex equipment, or patient fatigue related problem.

5. Prescription of Dose

5.1. Dose Prescription Values for TSEB

Prescribed dose in total skin electron beam therapy depends on disease staging and TSEB protocol variety. Bibliographically, TSEB irradiation doses range from 2.5 Gy to 42.5 Gy. The majority of radiotherapy clinics recommend radiation doses of 27 to 40 Gy, tending towards to a 36 Gy prescription, fractionated throughout a 9-week high-dose rate treatment scheme (4 sessions per week).

It is a common practice, to interrupt sessions for a short period (e.g. a week), and then resume treatment. Daily dose to skin ranges from 1 to 2 Gy. Occasionally, doses can reach up to 3 Gy or 4 Gy under the condition that time interval between two treatment sessions is one or two weeks, respectively [38].

5.2. Dose Prescription Point and Calibration Point

The delivery of the treatment dose is prescribed at the surface of the skin at the height of umbilicus of the patient (dose prescription point). Any dose value that is acquired by any dosimetric means on skin is normalized to this certain point. This spot should not be confused with the calibration point, which is located on the center of the stationary electron field (normally coincides with the umbilicus) at depth of maximum dose deposition (z_{max}). The ratio of the dose at calibration point to the corresponding dose at the prescription point (usually referred with the letter b) is a TSEB non-dimensional quality factor that indicates the influence of all contributing electron fields to total dose deposited on the patient. The b correlation is determined experimentally by phantom measurements during establishment process.

5.3. Boost Fields

Malignant regions of skin, which did not receive the whole amount of the prescribed dose (vertex, soles, axillaries, perineum, etc.), after the completion of TSEB sessions should be post-irradiated. Additional boost fields should be applied regionally, as in common electron therapies, using electron applicators and a conventional on-couch patient setup [72]. Depending on the remaining disease and area, pertinent literature suggests a 4 Gy to 26 Gy boost dose prescription range. To avoid supplementary irradiation courses in the scalp, some practitioners have adapted a lead reflector system over patient's vertex to enhance dose delivery during TSEB [11, 64]. The angle of the reflector is calculated individually for each patient in relation to his height and the amount of supplementary doses needed for the vertex.

6. Prescribed Dose Delivery Times: A Critical Treatment Quality Factor

Total skin electron beam therapy is quite a time-consuming procedure. Each treatment session duration could surpass a two-hour time period [16], including patient preparation, positioning and beam-on time. In addition, the feeble condition or even the age of a patient could rise the required time per session to unacceptable levels for the normal running of the clinical program. Extended source-skin distance increases required time of dose delivery, as the electron beam spreads in function to the distance and thus electron fluence is reduced. Therefore, performing a TSEB therapy with dose rates that are applied at routine radiation treatments (about 240 MU per minute) could end up to improper session delays, for a fully occupied radiation therapy department. Increased session time also affects the quality of the provided treatment, especially if the delay concerns time of dose delivery. Involuntary movements of a standing patient could lead to amplified dose heterogeneity all over the skin surface. The effect of patient motion is more intense in techniques that require standing patients. On top, a low dose rate protocol increases the possibility of patient dislocation of the original place of treatment.

Generally, rotational TSEB techniques provide the advantage of reduced daily beam-on time in comparison with other standing-patient techniques, due to the synchronized irradiation and rotation of the patient. Moreover, the total number of treatment sessions is halved, as the full coverage of the skin area is ensured in every session by the complete rotation of the patient. Nevertheless, the phase of rotation can be a torturous procedure for an aged and already physically burdened patient.

Therefore, time reducing of daily TSEB performance is a matter of major importance. To minimize required beam-on times, dose is delivered normally with a high dose rate of an average of 2500 MU per minute at the isocenter at the depth of maximum dose deposition from a single electron beam (z_{max}) [15, 17, 43]. The medical staff should be cognizant of the hazards that such a dose rate encompasses. Typically, in linear accelerators, which offer a high dose rate option, passwords and/or other interlocks almost preclude the likelihood of human error during treatment [43].

Anyhow, high dose rates ensure faster treatments. For an experienced team in a TSEB procedure, a linear accelerator, functioning on a high dose rate mode, could be occupied for a total skin irradiation session for an average time of 9.5 minutes [17] for rotational techniques or 15 minutes for a six dual-field protocol [16].

7. Safety Aspects and Precautions

Total skin electron beam therapy is, actually, a rather unconventional irradiation treatment. In contrast to any other radiation therapy, no treatment planning system (TPS) is utilized for the calculation of required Monitor Units and the beam-patient arrangement. This fact inserts great uncertainty regarding patient safety and therapy effectiveness. Thus, physicists should pay extra attention during the installation treatment and the design of clinical performance.

7.1. Field Dose Profile

A crucial physical parameter that should be determined precisely is the dose profile of the clinical electron field at the treatment plane. Regardless of the applied technique, the combination of two or more individual fields to produce a larger homogeneous field is the most sensitive parameter in TSEB establishment.

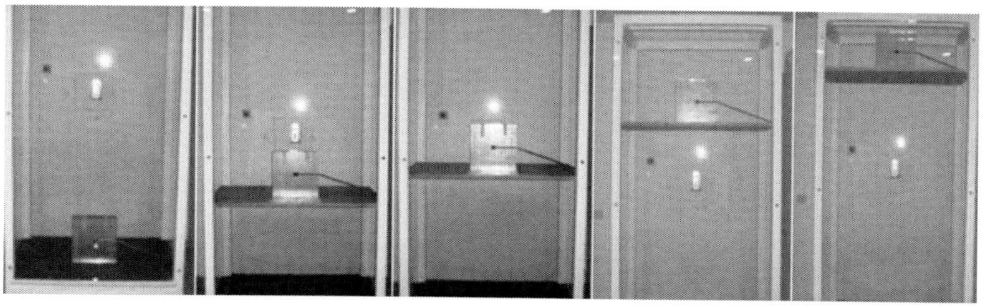

Figure 13. Indicative positions of experimental setup for the measurement of flatness and symmetry of the stationary electron field across the longitudinal axis.

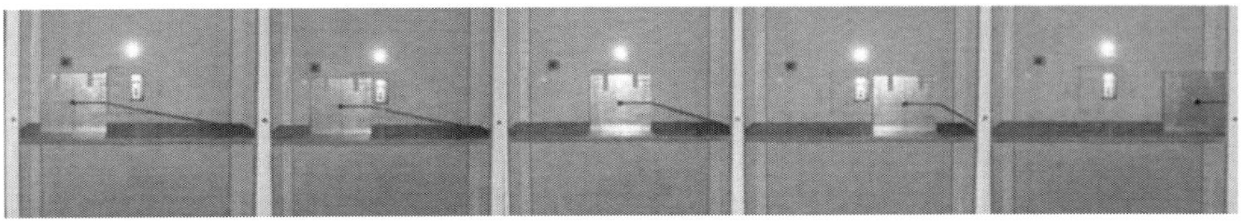

Figure 14. Indicative positions of experimental setup for the measurement of flatness and symmetry of the stationary electron field across the vertical axis.

For angled beam techniques, relative angle between component fields should be reconfirmed on a regular basis. Field dose profile should be measured along vertical and horizontal axis of treatment plane, focusing chiefly in field junction areas. Particular measurement protocols are essential, as the dimensions of clinical fields often exceed 200 x 80 cm^2 (Figure 13 and Figure 14).

7.2. Energy and Shape Modulation of Incident Electron Rays

Energy degrading of the beam is another factor that requires cautiously conducted measurements. The most probable energy (E_p) of electrons at the treatment plane for superficial irradiation should value about 4 MeV. In most linear accelerators, the 6 MeV option is the lowest accessible electron energy. As far as short-SSD techniques are concerned, intervening air layers are not sufficient to reduce electrons' initial energy adequately. Therefore, the utilization of tissue-equivalent screens (decelerators) is indicated [6]. Materials like PMMA, Perspex, Lucite, and Lexan, in the form of large sheets of appropriate thickness, are commonly interjected vertically to the pathway of the electron beam. Besides the desired energy degrading, these acrylic layers scatter as well incident electrons. This results in improved field flatness (and, consequently, better dose uniformity on patient) and slightly enlarged field dimensions. In some cases, when electron field flatness is not satisfactory, flattening filters made of aluminium, titanium and acrylic materials are attached to the beam's exit window on the head of the linear accelerator. Their shape and thickness are either experimentally determined or "in-silico" designed by the utilization of Monte Carlo simulation, in order to modulate properly field profile, without increasing an unacceptable X-ray background [19, 50].

7.3. Dose Homogeneity

A moderately homogeneous electron field at the treatment plane can be produced by all previously outlined techniques, if careful measurements have been carried out. Nevertheless, dose homogeneity on skin is a far more difficult objective. The human figure is an imponderable parameter even if a perfectly flattened field is applied on it. Furthermore, oblique incidence of electrons at the various treatment postures could cause unpredictable dose distribution. The ±5% average field uniformity limit (see §2.1.3) can be turned into a threefold dose inhomogeneity on the skin of the patient. Effectively, in all bibliographically referred TSEB techniques, observed average dose homogeneity exhibits average variations from up to ±15% [1, 9, 66]. Better dose distribution can be presented mostly at flattened areas of the body such as the patient's trunk surface. In other regions of the body, anatomical folds can alter dose distribution underneath them and cause significant underdosage. Dose uniformity can also be affected by scattered electrons from the material of the floor, directed mainly towards the legs of the patient. The performance of techniques that irradiation occurs simultaneously with relative motion of patient (rotational, translational, etc), requires constant mechanical tests of motor stability and speed reproducibility to avoid undesirable complications in skin dose distribution.

7.4. Bremsstrahlung Contaminating Photons

Avoiding superfluous X-ray photons, resulting to skin, is another major TSEB challenge [6, 10, 33]. The production of X-rays is a result of electron interactions with the parts of the head of the linear accelerator and the assisting equipment. This phenomenon depends on the energy of electrons, the atomic number (Z) and the thickness of the materials. Generally, the contribution of accompanying X-rays to the total dose absorbed by the patient is approximately proportional to the number of constituent electron fields [6]. Angled beam techniques offer a solution to this problem by directing the greater percentage of redundant Bremsstrahlung radiation outwards the body. The -xray background also seems to be affected by the distance of the decelerator from the electron source. Materials close to the head produce more intense X-rays comparable to larger degraders placed near the treatment plane [6].

Variations of the Bremsstrahlung intensity are obtained along the dimensions of the clinical field. At the horizontal axis, at every applied technique, the intensity reaches its maximum value at the center of the axis, and then progressively degrades to the edge of the field. On the contrary, at the longitudinal axis, the variations seem to be technique-dependent. In case of single field irradiation techniques, photon distribution resembles vertical axis intensity behavior. If a multiple angle field technique is applied, then the maximum value of intensity is located at near the edges of the clinical field, around the central axis of the angled beams, while moving towards the field center, Bremsstrahlung contribution declines.

The guidelines of AAPM suggest that the percentage of contamination photons should be kept under 4% (this percentage is interpreted to about 1.5 Gy of the total dose absorbed by TSEB procedure) [6]. In the relevant literature, contamination from Bremsstrahlung photons ranges from 2.7% [15] to the maximum percentage of 5% [14], with rotational techniques offering, in general, lower X-ray exposure in total.

8. An Example of TSEB Treatment Installation and Performance

In our radiation therapy unit, a Total Skin Electron beam therapy technique was established [11]. A six dual-field setup was designed, based on the special technical features of the existing treatment room. The final choice of the utilized technique was made after a series of experiments and individual (room and patient associated) parameter determination. The linear accelerator used is a Clinac 2100C (Varian, Palo Alto, California, US) with the capability of producing five nominal electron beam energies, within the spectrum of 6 MeV to 21 MeV. In addition, the linear accelerator was calibrated to provide two total skin electron beam modes of low and high dose delivery rate, respectively. The second one was preferred for practical reasons. No electron applicator was utilized for beam formation. Instead, a dedicated TSEB tray was inserted into the special holder of the head of the linear accelerator. The purpose of the tray is to automatically adjust all parameters of the linear accelerator to clinical high dose rate TSEB mode. Energy is set at 6 MeV (in order to achieve superficial energy deposition), collimators form a field of 36 x 36 cm^2 at the isocenter, and dose rate reaches its maximum value, which is 2500 MU per minute. A hand-crafted immobilization system is placed in the room, opposite to the head of the accelerator. The system is portable, placed on top of five wheels, securely attached to the floor and capable of bearing the weight of at least 300 kilograms. It is lifted about 25 cm from the ground to decrease the percentage of the scattered-to-floor electrons directed to skin. Its dimensions are sufficiently large for a person to stand in it. In the interior, two long straps are hanging from the top, in order to support the standing patient, and allow him to take in total, six positions of treatment.

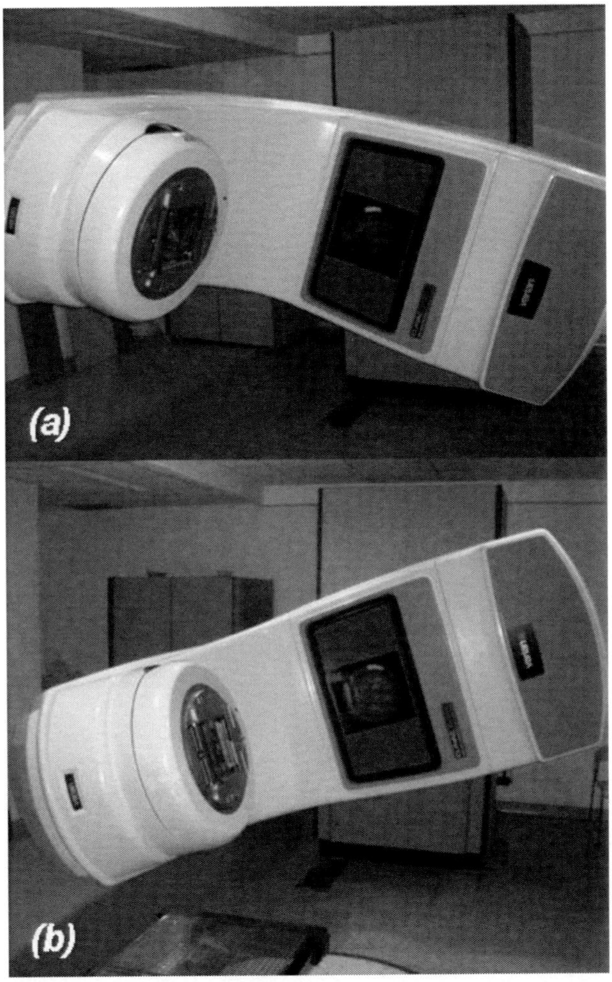

Figure 15. Successive irradiation positions of the linear accelerator in order to achieve a large and homogenous electron field at treatment plane (SSD = 380 cm) (a) 252.5° (b) 287.5° degrees.

In the side that faces the linear accelerator, a large PMMA sheet, with a thickness of 0.5cm, is attached. The appropriate value of the thickness was calculated experimentally to reduce the energy of the incident electrons to almost 3.4 MeV on the skin surface. Additionally, the acrylic sheet scatters electrons and homogenates the clinical field. For certain cases, when the scalp of the patient requires extra dose delivery, a 0.4cm lead reflector is placed above the head of the patient at specific (patient and dose dependent) angles. The distance between the outer surface of the PMMA layer and the isocenter of the accelerator is 250cm, while the umbilicus of the patient should always be located 30cm distant from the inner surface of the PMMA layer. Hence, source-skin distance is 380cm. The gantry of the linear accelerator takes two angles of irradiation, per treatment position. Field flatness is the basic criterion for the choice of the proper gantry angle, which, in our case, was achieved by the combination of 272.5^{o} and 287.5^{o} degrees gantry positions (tilt of $\pm 17.5^{o}$ degrees from the horizontal position of the gantry) (Figure 15). The patient stands in the immobilization system, and takes six positions, with 60° degrees angular shift from each other (Figure 9). At each position, he stands with a distinct posture, trying to reveal as much as possible surface of his body (Figure 16).

Prescribed dose is normally about 36 Gy in total, and it is fractionated to 4 Gy per week. Each day, only three out of six treatment positions are performed, resulting in a 2 Gy per 2 days dose absorption to skin. Throughout treatment, the uniformity of doses on patients is mapped utilizing thermoluminescence dosemeters, calibrated for total skin irradiation conditions. The average dose homogeneity in our patients is repeatable and varies among ±7% to ±12% (normalized to the dose received by the skin at umbilicus), depending mostly on the body figure of the patient (Figure 17). Bremsstrahlung photons maximum percentage, located at the upper and lower edges of the TSEB field, was 2.1% of the total dose delivered to patient.

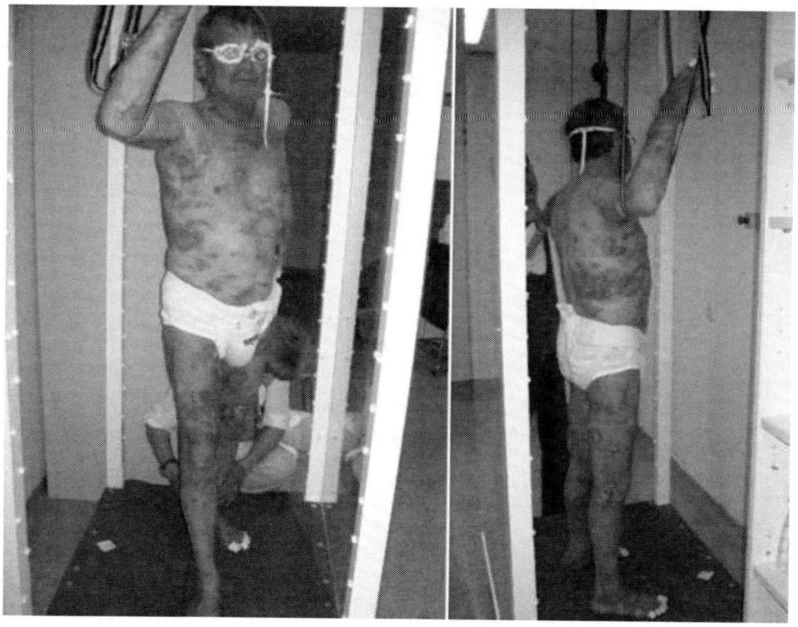

Figure 16. Patient preparation and positioning on the immobilization system before the initiation of a treatment session. Lead shielding is applied on his eyes, genitals and the nails of his hands and toes.

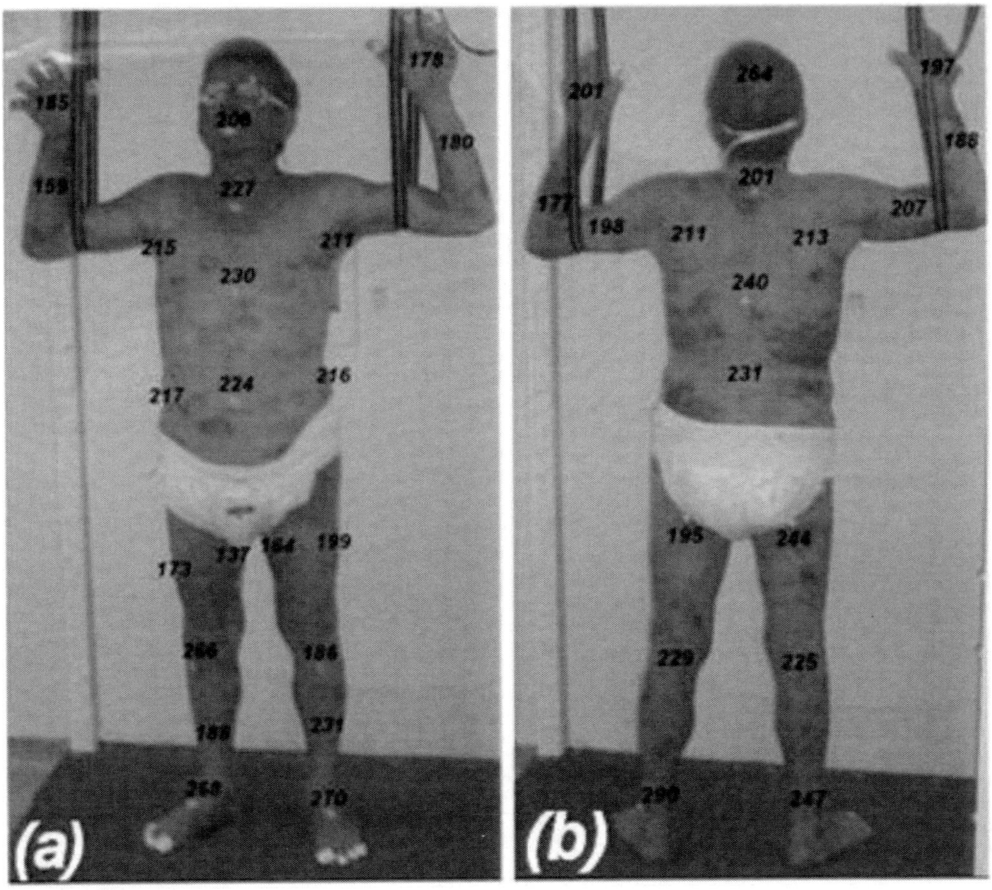

Figure 17. Dose distribution (absolute values expressed in cGy) on the surface of the patient after the completion of a six dual-field irradiation cycle. Dose values were obtained by thermoluminescent dosimeters (TLDs) distributed all over skin. (a) Anterior surface dose distribution (b) Posterior surface dose distribution.

At every session, and according to the dose prescribed by the radiation oncologist, personalized lead shields protect the sensitive areas of the body. Eyes, nails, and genitals are covered at every session. After receiving an amount of 20 Gy, the scalp of the head is shielded as well, intending to reduce as much as possible the inevitable irradiation-originated alopecia. Underdosed areas mainly appeared in neck, armpits, bubonic area and gluteal creases.

On the other hand, feet are usually overdosed, due to the electrons that are scattered from the material of the floor and result on patient. Radiation side effects are present throughout the treatment procedure. Skin responds acutely to absorbed doses.

Erythema, edema, wet desquamation, bleeding, local pruritus, and fatigue are common side effects that patients have to endure during the period of irradiation. The benefits from the treatment are usually observed after one month since the performance of the last TSEB treatment (Figure 18, Figure 19, and Figure 20).

Areas of the body that resist treatment, and remain malignant, are treated by an additional course of boost electron fields. The supplementary dose is delivered regionally by the conventional 6 MeV electron therapy mode.

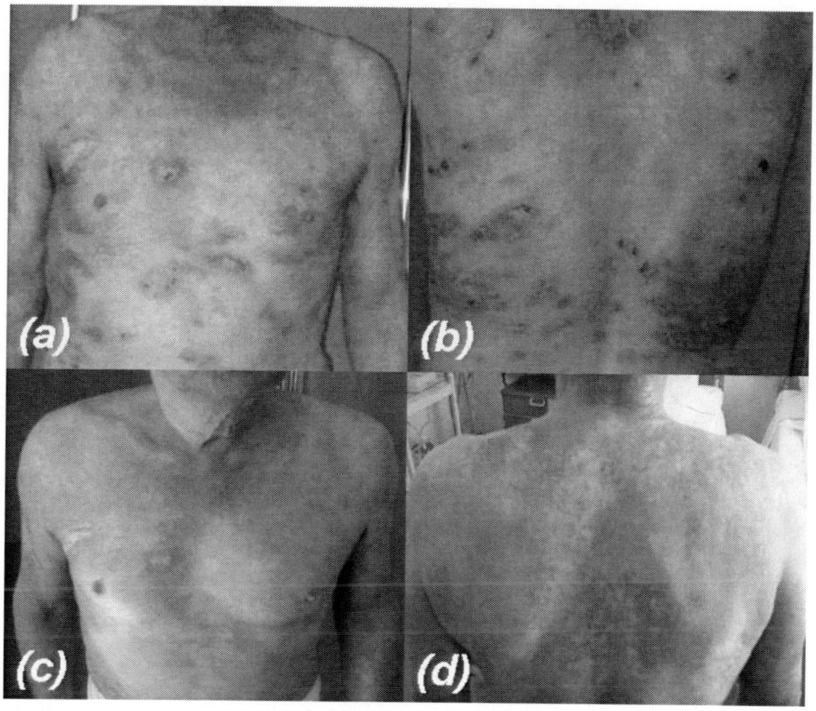

Figure 18. TSEB efficacy for a Mycosis Fungoides patient. Condition of (a) chest skin and (b) back skin before receiving treatment. Condition of (c) chest skin and (d) back skin one month after the end of the irradiation procedure.

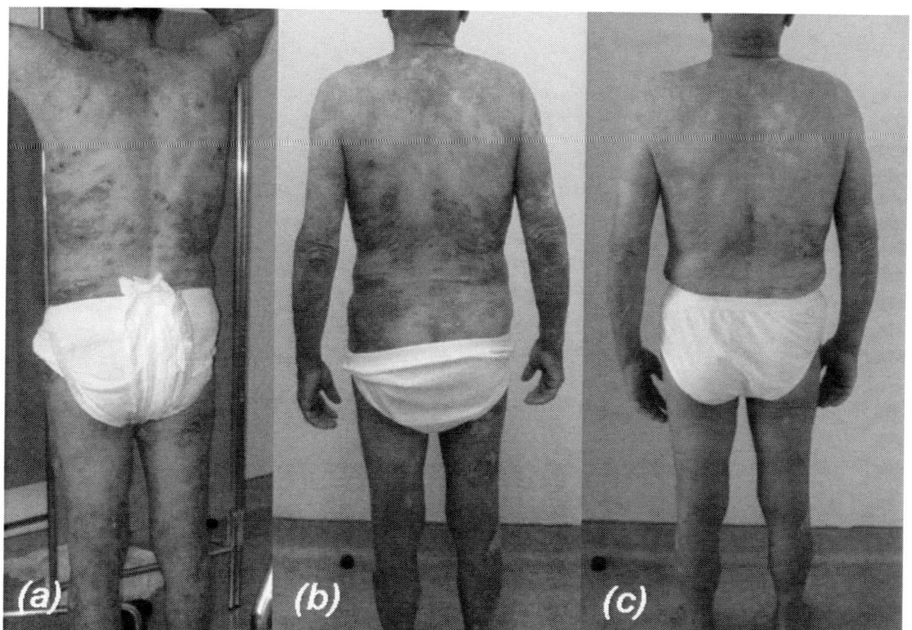

Figure 19. Progressive improvement of clinical condition of a Mycosis Fungoides patient that received TSEB treatment (Prescribed dose = 36 Gy). (a) At the beginning of the irradiations (b) right after the last TSEB session (c) one month after the last session.

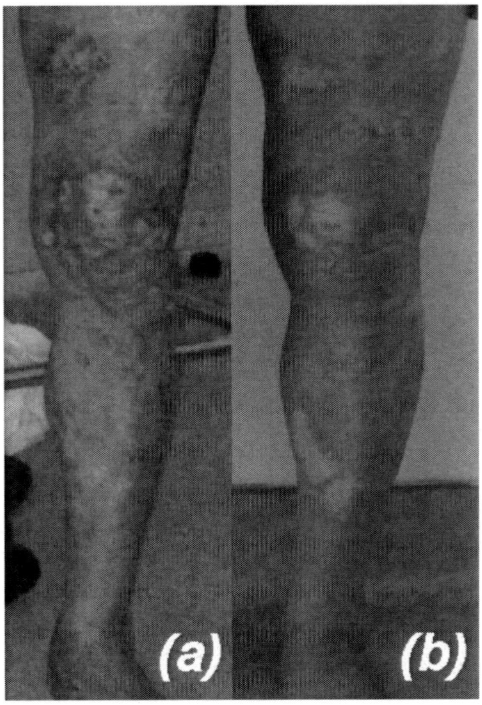

Figure 20. Clinical condition of the left leg of a Mycosis Fungoides patient (a) before the first TSEB session (b) one month after the last TSEB session.

CONCLUSION

Total skin electron beam irradiation is a successful tool in the management of cutaneous T-cell lymphoma. TSEB efficacy is attributed to the physical properties of high-energy electrons. Either as monotherapy or supplementary treatment, the prescription of TSEB treatment could lead even to complete remission of the disease symptoms, particularly for patients of early stage lymphoma. Carefully designed shielding equipment in combination to a high dose rate protocol could restrict the inevitable radiation toxicity side effects. Special attention should be paid to designing and carrying out frequently a quality assurance program, related to TSEB procedure exclusively. Although the basic prerequisite to implement a TSEB technique is an electron beam providing linear accelerator (and enough space in the room of treatment), only a limited number of health centers worldwide administers this treatment, due to its complexity. Existent variety in TSEB performance is an outcome of the effort to match the discrete characteristics of each clinic with patient comfort. The vast majority of radiation therapy centers have ended up using the "six dual-field" TSEB technique, which is founded on an irradiation method developed by Stanford University in the early 1970's. Dose prescription is disease-stage dependent, and varies according to the technique selected by the medical physicist and the radiation oncologist. An indicated prescription dose range is from 36 Gy to 40 Gy. The total amount of dose is commonly fractionated to 4 Gy per week for 9 weeks with or without interval. "Self-shielded" anatomical sites of body that did not treated sufficiently, are spotted by "in vivo" dosimetry. The remaining dose is delivered to them, by the prescription of locally administered electron fields.

REFERENCES

[1] Funk, A., Hensley F., Krempien R., Neuhof D., Van Kampen M., Treiber M., et al. Palliative total skin electron beam therapy (TSEBT) for advanced cutaneous T-cell lymphoma. *Eur. J. Dermatol.,* 2008: 18(3); 308-12.

[2] Lansigan, F., Choi, J., Foss, F.M. Cutaneous T-cell lymphoma. *Hematol. Oncol. Clin. North Am.,* 2008: 22(5); 979-96, x.

[3] Wilcox, R.A. Cutaneous T-cell lymphoma: 2011 update on diagnosis, risk-stratification, and management. *Am. J. Hematol.* 86(11); 928-48.

[4] Trump, J.G., Webster, E.W., Wright, K.A., Evans, W.W., Granke, R.C., Hare, H.F., et al. Physical and clinical aspects of supervoltage rotational therapy. *Radiology,* 1951: 57(2); 157-68.

[5] Andreo, P., Burns, D.T., Hohlfeld, K., Huq, M.S., Kanai, T., Laitano, F., et al. IAEA TRS-398: Absorbed Dose Determination in External Beam Radiotherapy: *An International Code of Practice for Dosimetry based on Standards of Absorbed Dose to Water,* ed. I.A.E. Agency-IAEA. Vol. 10. 2000.

[6] Karzmack, C.J., Anderson, J., Fessenden, P., Svensson, G., Buffa, A., Khan, F., et al. AAPM Report No.23, Total Skin Electron therapy: Technique and Dosimetry, Report of Group 30 *Radiation therapy Committee AAPM.* 1987.

[7] Podgorsak, E.B. Review of Radiaton Oncology Physics: *A Handbook for Teachers and Students,* ed. I.A.E. Agency. 2003, Vienna, Austria.

[8] Diamantopoulos, S., Platoni, K., Dilvoi, M., Nazos, I., Geropantas, K., Maravelis, G., et al. Clinical implementation of total skin electron beam (TSEB) therapy: a review of the relevant literature. *Phys. Med.* 27(2); 62-8.

[9] Chen, Z., Agostinelli A., Nath R. On the use of unshielded cables in ionization chamber dosimetry for total-skin electron therapy. *Phy.s Med. Biol.,* 1998: 43(3); 539-46.

[10] Das, I.J., Copeland, J.F., Bushe, H.S. Spatial distribution of bremsstrahlung in a dual electron beam used in total skin electron treatments: errors due to ionization chamber cable irradiation. *Med. Phys.,* 1994: 21(11); 1733-8.

[11] Platoni, K., Diamantopoulos, S., Panayiotakis, G., Kouloulias, V., Pantelakos, P., Kelekis, N., et al. First application of total skin electron beam irradiation in Greece: setup, measurements and dosimetry. *Phys. Med.* 28(2); 174-82.

[12] Gamble, L.M., Farrell, T.J., Jones, G.W., Hayward, J.E. Two-dimensional mapping of underdosed areas using radiochromic film for patients undergoing total skin electron beam radiotherapy. *Int. J. Radiat. Oncol. Biol. Phys.,* 2005: 62(3); 920-4.

[13] Antolak, J.A., Cundiff, J.H., Ha, C.S. Utilization of thermoluminescent dosimetry in total skin electron beam radiotherapy of mycosis fungoides. *Int. J. Radiat. Oncol. Biol. Phys.,* 1998: 40(1); 101-8.

[14] Shouman, T., El-Taher, Z. Total skin electron therapy: a modified technique for small room linear accelerator. *J. Egypt Natl. Canc. Inst.,* 2004: 16(4); 202-9.

[15] Reynard, E.P., Evans, M.D., Devic, S., Parker, W., Freeman, C.R., Roberge, D., et al. Rotational total skin electron irradiation with a linear accelerator. *J. Appl. Clin. Med. Phys.,* 2008: 9(4); 2793.

[16] Parida, D.K., Verma, K.K., Chander, S., Joshi, R.C., Rath, G.K. Total skin electron irradiation therapy in mycosis fungoides using high-dose rate mode: a preliminary experience. *Int. J. Dermatol.,* 2005: 44(10); 828-30.

[17] Evans, M.O., Seuntjens, J., Parker, W., Devic, S., Poli, E., Freeman, C., Podgorsak, E. SU-FF-T-387: *Rotational Total Skin Electron Irradiation Using a Commercially Available Linear Accelerator with a High Dose Rate Total Body Electron Mode Medical Physics*, 2006: 33(6); 2134-5.

[18] Wu, J.M., Leung, S.W., Wang, C.J., Chui, C.S. Lying-on position of total skin electron therapy. *Int. J. Radiat. Oncol. Biol. Phys.*, 1997: 39(2); 521-8.

[19] Ye, S.J., Pareek, P.N., Spencer, S., Duan, J., Brezovich, I.A. Monte Carlo techniques for scattering foil design and dosimetry in total skin electron irradiations. *Med. Phys.*, 2005: 32(6); 1460-8.

[20] Turner, J.R., Hugtenburg, R.P., Wynne, C.J. Total skin electron therapy at two energies on a linear accelerator. *Australas. Phys. Eng. Sci. Med.,* 1995: 18(4); 208-20.

[21] Quiros, P.A., Jones, G.W., Kacinski, B.M., Braverman, I.M., Heald, P.W., Edelson, R.L., et al. Total skin electron beam therapy followed by adjuvant psoralen/ultraviolet-A light in the management of patients with T1 and T2 cutaneous T-cell lymphoma (mycosis fungoides). *Int. J. Radiat. Oncol. Biol. Phys.*, 1997: 38(5); 1027-35.

[22] Jones, G.W., Wilson L.D. Mycosis fungoides and total skin electron beam radiation. *Blood,* 1997: 89(8); 3062-4.

[23] Weaver, R.D., Gerbi, B.J., Dusenbery, K.E., Evaluation of dose variation during total skin electron irradiation using thermoluminescent dosimeters. *Int. J. Radiat. Oncol. Biol. Phys.*, 1995: 33(2); 475-8.

[24] Peters, V.G., Jaywant, S.M. Implementation of total skin electron therapy using an optional high dose rate mode on a conventional linear accelerator. *Med. Dosim.*, 1995: 20(2); 99-104.

[25] el-Khatib, E.G., Rymel, J., al-Mokhlef J. A technique for total skin electron irradiation using six large flattened electron beams: implementation on linear accelerators having different modes of electron beam production. *Br. J. Radiol.*, 1989: 62(740); 744-8.

[26] Earley, L., Moeller, J., O'Rear, J., Leavitt, D.D. A method for total skin electron treatment for infants. *Med Dosim*, 1995: 20(4); 243-8.

[27] Strohl, R.A. The role of total skin electron beam radiation therapy in the management of mycosis fungoides. *Dermatol. Nurs.*, 1994: 6(3); 191-4, 6, 220.

[28] Kuten, A., Stein, M., Mandelzweig, Y., Tatcher, M., Yaacov, G., Epelbaum, R., et al. Total-skin electron irradiation for cutaneous T-cell lymphoma: the Northern Israel Oncology Center experience. *Strahlenther. Onkol.*, 1991: 167(7); 392-6.

[29] Kuten, A., Rosenblatt, E., Dale, J., Leviov, M., Tatcher, M. Total skin electron irradiation: efficacy in early mycosis fungoides. *Leuk. Lymphoma*, 1993: 10(4-5); 281-5.

[30] Van Der Merwe, D.G. Total skin electron therapy: a technique which can be implemented on a conventional electron linear accelerator. *Int. J. Radiat. Oncol. Biol. Phys.*, 1993: 27(2); 391-6.

[31] Freeman, C.R., Suissa, S., Shenouda, G., Vuong, T., Souhami, L., Pla M., et al. Clinical experience with a single field rotational total skin electron irradiation technique for cutaneous T-cell lymphoma. *Radiother. Oncol.,* 1992: 24(3); 155-62.

[32] Hoppe, R.T. Total skin electron beam therapy in the management of mycosis fungoides. *Front. Radiat. Ther. Oncol.*, 1991: 25; 80-9; discussion 132-3.

[33] el-Khatib, E.E., Scrimger, J., Murray, B., Reduction of the Bremsstrahlung component of clinical electron beams: implications for electron arc therapy and total skin electron irradiation. *Phys. Med. Biol.,* 1991: 36(1); 111-8.

[34] Cox, R.S., Heck, R.J., Fessenden, P., Karzmark, C.J., Rust, D.C. Development of total-skin electron therapy at two energies. *Int. J. Radiat. Oncol. Biol. Phys.,* 1990: 18(3); 659-69.

[35] Chinn, D.M., Chow, S., Kim, Y.H., Hoppe, R.T. Total skin electron beam therapy with or without adjuvant topical nitrogen mustard or nitrogen mustard alone as initial treatment of T2 and T3 mycosis fungoides. *Int. J. Radiat. Oncol. Biol. Phys.*, 1999: 43(5); 951-8.

[36] Antolak, J.A., Hogstrom K.R. Multiple scattering theory for total skin electron beam design. *Med. Phys.,* 1998: 25(6); 851-9.

[37] Leung, S.W., Hsu, H.C., Huang, P.H. Total skin electron beam irradiation in scleromyxoedema. *Br. J. Radiol.,* 1998: 71(841); 84-6.

[38] Rosenblatt, E., Kuten, A., Leviov, M., Cederbaum, M. Total skin electron irradiation in mycosis fungoides dose and fractionation considerations. *Leuk. Lymphoma*, 1998: 30(1-2); 143-51.

[39] Jones, G.W., Rosenthal, D., Wilson, L.D. Total skin electron radiation for patients with erythrodermic cutaneous T-cell lymphoma (mycosis fungoides and the Sezary syndrome). *Cancer*, 1999: 85(9); 1985-95.

[40] R. Ravichandran, K.K., Sivakumar, S.S., Davis, C.A., Mohanti, B.K. Clinical electron beam configuration and physical parameters for total skin electron treatment (TSET). *Journal of Medical Physics*, 2005: 30(2).

[41] Corvo, R., Giudici, S., Maggio, F., Bevegni, M., Sampietro, C., Lucido, M.R., et al. Weekly concomitant boost in adjuvant radiotherapy for patients with early breast cancer: preliminary results on feasibility. *Tumori,* 2008: 94(5); 706-11.

[42] Ulutin, H.C., Beyan, C., Pak, Y. Total skin electron beam therapy for cutaneous T-cell lymphoma: Turkish experience with translational technique. *Hematologia (Budap),* 2002: 32(4); 397-403.

[43] Parida, D.K., Verma, K.K., Rath, G.K., Total skin electron irradiation treatment for mycosis fungoides with a new alternate daily treatment schedule to minimize radiation-associated toxicity: a preliminary experience. *Clin. Exp. Dermatol.,* 2009: 34(5); e37-9.

[44] Pepek, J.M., Paulino, A.C., Briones, M.A., Marcus, R.B., Jr., Esiashvili N. Role of total skin electron beam therapy for leukemia cutis in pediatric patients. *Pediatr. Blood Cancer,* 2008: 50(5); 1054-5.

[45] Kamstrup, M.R., Specht, L., Skovgaard, G.L., Gniadecki, R. A prospective, open-label study of low-dose total skin electron beam therapy in mycosis fungoides. *Int. J. Radiat. Oncol. Biol. Phys.,* 2008: 71(4); 1204-7.

[46] Introcaso, C.E., Micaily, B., Richardson, S.K., Junkins-Hopkins, J.M., Yoon, J.S., Kim, E.J., et al. Total skin electron beam therapy may be associated with improvement of peripheral blood disease in Sezary syndrome. *J. Am. Acad. Dermatol.,* 2008: 58(4); 592-5.

[47] Bufacchi, A., Carosi, A., Adorante, N., Delle Canne, S., Malatesta, T., Capparella, R., et al. In vivo EBT radiochromic film dosimetry of electron beam for Total Skin Electron Therapy (TSET). *Phys. Med.,* 2007: 23(2); 67-72.

[48] Ravichandran, M.R.A.R. Measurement of physical parameters for total skin electron therapy with a medial accelerator. *Journal of Medical Physics,* 1999: 24(1).

[49] Quinlan, K.E., Janiga, J.J., Baran, R., Lim H.W. Transverse melanonychia secondary to total skin electron beam therapy: a report of 3 cases. *J. Am. Acad. Dermatol.,* 2005: 53(2 Suppl 1); S112-4.

[50] Pham, Y.T., Bubb, I.F., Cramb, J.A. Electron scattering filter design for a single field rotational total skin irradiation. *Australas Phys. Eng. Sci. Med.,* 2005: 28(3); 145-50.

[51] K. Krishnamurthy, C.A.D., Ravichandran, R., Sivakumar, S.S., Mohanti, B.K. Radiaton dose delivery for total skin electron therapy (TSET) with low energy electron beams. *Journal of Medical Physics,* 2005: 30(2).

[52] Reavely, M.M., Wilson, L.D. Total skin electron beam therapy and cutaneous T-cell lymphoma: a clinical guide for patients and staff. *Dermatol. Nurs.,* 2004: 16(1); 36, 9, 57.

[53] Piermattei, A., Rossi, G., Azario, L., Fidanzio, A., Balducci, M., Valentini V. Electron beam dosimetry of Total Skin Electron Therapy (TSET). *Radiol. Med.,* 2004: 108(5-6); 549-59.

[54] Gossman, M.S., Sharma S.C. Total skin high-dose-rate electron therapy dosimetry using TG-51. *Med. Dosim.,* 2004: 29(4); 285-7.

[55] Chen, Z., Agostinelli, A.G., Wilson, L.D., Nath, R. Matching the dosimetry characteristics of a dual-field Stanford technique to a customized single-field Stanford technique for total skin electron therapy. *Int. J. Radiat. Oncol. Biol. Phys.*, 2004: 59(3); 872-85.

[56] Wilson, L.D. Delivery and sequelae of total skin electron beam therapy. *Arch. Dermatol.,* 2003: 139(6); 812-3.

[57] Smith, B.D., Son, C.B., Wilson, L.D. Disseminated herpes simplex after total skin electron beam radiotherapy for mycosis fungoides. *J. R. Soc. Med.,* 2003: 96(10); 500-1.

[58] Piotrowski, T., Fundowicz, D., Pawlaczyk, M., Malicki J. Thermoluminescent dosimetry in rotary-dual technique of the total skin electron irradiation. *Neoplasma,* 2003: 50(2); 125-30.

[59] Pavon, E.C., Sanchez-Doblado, F., Leal, A., Capote, R., Lagares, J.I., Perucha, M., et al. Total skin electron therapy treatment verification: Monte Carlo simulation and beam characteristics of large non-standard electron fields. *Phys. Med. Biol.,* 2003: 48(17); 2783-96.

[60] Jones, G., Wilson, L.D., Fox-Goguen, L. Total skin electron beam radiotherapy for patients who have mycosis fungoides. *Hematol. Oncol. Clin. North. Am.,* 2003: 17(6); 1421-34.

[61] Gamble, L.M., Farrell, T.J., Jones, G.W., Hayward, J.E. Composite depth dose measurement for total skin electron (TSE) treatments using radiochromic film. *Phys. Med. Biol.,* 2003: 48(7); 891-8.

[62] Maingon, P., Truc, G., Dalac, S., Barillot, I., Lambert, D., Petrella, T., et al. Radiotherapy of advanced mycosis fungoides: indications and results of total skin electron beam and photon beam irradiation. *Radiother. Oncol.,* 2000: 54(1); 73-8.
[63] Wilson, L.D., Jones, G.W., Kim, D., Rosenthal, D., Christensen, I.R., Edelson, R.L., et al. Experience with total skin electron beam therapy in combination with extracorporeal photopheresis in the management of patients with erythrodermic (T4) mycosis fungoides. *J. Am. Acad. Dermatol.,* 2000: 43(1 Pt 1); 54-60.
[64] Peters, V.G. Use of an electron reflector to improve dose uniformity at the vertex during total skin electron therapy. *Int. J. Radiat. Oncol. Biol. Phys.,* 2000: 46(4); 1065-9.
[65] Anacak, Y., Arican, Z., Drumea, K., Rosenblatt, E., Tamir, A., Chetver, L., et al. Total skin electron irradiation in mycosis fungoides: comparison between a modified Christie Hospital translational technique and the Stanford technique. *Leuk. Lymphoma,* 2002: 43(11); 2093-7.
[66] Anacak, Y., Arican, Z., Bar-Deroma, R., Tamir, A., Kuten, A. Total skin electron irradiation: evaluation of dose uniformity throughout the skin surface. *Med. Dosim.,* 2003: 28(1); 31-4.
[67] Jones, G.W., Kacinski, B.M., Wilson, L.D., Willemze, R., Spittle, M., Hohenberg, G., et al. Total skin electron radiation in the management of mycosis fungoides: Consensus of the European Organization for Research and Treatment of Cancer (EORTC) Cutaneous Lymphoma Project Group. *J. Am. Acad. Dermatol.,* 2002: 47(3); 364-70.
[68] Rampino, M., Ragona, R., Monetti, U., Mussano, A., Guarneri, A., Sannazzari, G.L. Total skin electron beam therapy in mycosis fungoides. Our experience from 1985 to 1999. *Radiol. Med.,* 2002: 103(1-2); 108-14.
[69] Margaretic, D., Faj, D., Tomas, I., Dmitrovic, B., Krajina, Z. Total skin electron treatment of extensive cutaneous lesions in Kaposi sarcoma. *Croat. Med. J.,* 2002: 43(3); 342-5.
[70] Faj, D., Vrtar, M., Krajina, Z., Jurkovic, S., Margaretic, D. Model of total skin electron treatment using the 'six-dual-field' technique. *Coll. Antropol.,* 2003: 27(2); 713-21
[71] Trump, J.G., Wright, K.A., Evans, W.W., Anson, J.H., Hare, H.F., Fromer, J.L., et al. High energy electrons for the treatment of extensive superficial malignant lesions. *Am. J. Roentgenol. Radium. Ther. Nucl. Med.,* 1953: 69(4); 623-9.
[72] Wilson, L.D., Quiros, P.A., Kolenik, S.A., Heald, P.W., Braverman, I.M., Edelson, R.L., et al. Additional courses of total skin electron beam therapy in the treatment of patients with recurrent cutaneous T-cell lymphoma. *J. Am. Acad. Dermatol.,* 1996: 35(1); 69-73.

In: Hodgkin's and T-Cell Lymphoma
Editors: Warren K. Harvey and Randall M. Jacobs
ISBN 978-1-62257-478-0

Chapter 3

HODGKIN'S DISEASE: EPIDEMIOLOGY, TREATMENT AND PROGNOSIS

Pinki K. Prasad
Louisiana State University Health Sciences Center,
Baton Rouge, LA, US

ABSTRACT

Hodgkin lymphoma (HL) is one of the most common malignancies in adolescents and older adults, accounting for more than 10% of the cancers annually in the developed world. It has a bimodal age distribution curve with the pattern of age incidence differing by geographic location. There are epidemiological risk factors that are associated with developing HL and they include family history of lymphoma, exposure to Epstein Barr virus, socioeconomic status, residence and social contacts. Hodgkin Lymphoma can be divided into two pathologic classes which include classical HL and nodular lymphocyte predominant HL. Clinically, most patients present with painless adenopathy and a constellation of systemic symptoms such as fever, weight loss, or night sweats that are considered B symptoms and are important for treatment and prognosis. Diagnosis of HL relies on a physical examination and history, computed topography scans along with newer nuclear medicine imaging fluorodeoxyglucose positron emission tomography (FDG-PET). Standard treatment includes risk adapted chemotherapy and radiotherapy. Treatment for recurrent or resistant disease includes conventional chemo and radiotherapy and hematopoietic stem cell transplant. Through prognosis remains very favorable with over 70% of patients being cured of their disease there are a number of adverse long term effects from therapy. Potential adverse long term toxicities can include cardiopulmonary dysfunction, gonadal dysfunction, infertility, thyroid disease and secondary malignancies. Modern era treatment aims to decrease toxicity from therapy while advancing the cure rate.

INTRODUCTION

Hodgkin lymphoma (HL), formerly called Hodgkin's disease, arises from germinal center or post-germinal center B cells. Hodgkin lymphoma is characterized by progressive enlargement of the lymph nodes. It is considered unicentric in origin and has a predictable pattern of spread by extension to contiguous nodes.

EPIDEMIOLOGY

Hodgkin lymphoma (HL) is one of the most common malignancies in adolescents and older adults, accounting for more than 10 percent of all lymphomas and approximately 0.6 percent of all cancers diagnosed in the developed world annually [1]. This amounts to approximately 9060 new cases and about 1190 deaths due to HL in the United States annually. It has a bimodal age distribution curve with the pattern of incidence differing by geographic location. In the US and other economically advantaged countries, HL has one peak at 15–35 years of age and the other above 50 years of age; though the incidence is highest among 15 to 19 year olds [2]. In economically disadvantaged areas, there is an initial peak in childhood for boys, relatively low rates in young adults, and a late peak in older adults. [3] There is a slight male predominance, especially in children and in middle and older adulthood.

Histology of HL also differs by age and gender. The most common histological subtype seen in the US and other developed countries is the nodular sclerosing subtype. The nodular sclerosing subtype (NSHL) is seen in over 70% of cases and is most commonly found in the adolescent and young adult population under the age of 20 years. In economically disadvantaged areas, mixed cellularity HL (MCHL) is more frequent in children and older adults. Early industrialized or transitional economies tend to have an equal frequency of MCHL and NSHL subtypes [4, 5].

RISK FACTORS

Several risk factors have been reported with an increase in risk of developing HL. These include family history of HL, Epstein Barr virus (EBV) infections, socioeconomic status and social contacts. Familial HL represents 4.5% of all HL cases. For adolescents and young adults there is a 99 fold increased risk among monozygotic twins and a 7 fold increased risk among siblings but not among older adults [6-8].

EBV has been most commonly reported with the mixed cellularity histologic subtype seen in children from underdeveloped countries and in young adult males. In young adult males, a history of infectious mononucleosis and high titer antibodies to EBV are associated with HL. EBV genetic material can be detected in Reed Sternberg (R-S) cells from some patients with HL.

There is an association between HL and socioeconomic status. In children less than 10 years of age, HL is associated with lower socioeconomic status and households with more children. However, in adolescents and individuals though middle adulthood, HL increased with higher socioeconomic status and with smaller households with fewer children [9,10]. Those individuals from industrially developed countries with higher socioeconomic status were more likely to develop the NSHL subtype. These findings may be related to an association with infections; increased infections in early childhood may decrease the risk of HL in young adults. In comparison, the risk pattern for the mixed cellularity HL (MCHL) subtype is inversely related to socioeconomic status [11]. Among lower socioeconomic groups in economically advantaged populations, cases of HL are predominantly of MCHL and lymphocytes depleted HL (LDHL) subtypes, and are more frequently Epstein Barr virus (EBV) positive [12].

Other risk factors include the increased risk of HL in those patients receiving immunosuppressive therapy. Patients that have received a solid organ transplant, hematopoietic stem cell transplant, or those on immunosuppressive therapy for autoimmune disorders or HIV infections have a higher incidence of HL than the normal population. [13-17] Most HL cases occurring in the setting of HIV infection are EBV-positive and many belong to the otherwise rare lymphocyte-depletion subtype.

Biology

The Reed Sternberg (R-S) cell is the hallmark of classical HL and is characterized by a binucleated or a multinucleated giant cell that is often characterized by a bilobed nucleus, with two large nucleoli, giving the classically described "owl's eye" appearance [18-20]. The R-S cells are embedded within a reactive infiltrate of lymphocytes, macrophages, granulocytes and eosinophils.

Reed Sternberg cells and its variants most commonly are derived from a neoplastic clone originating from B lymphocytes in lymph node germinal centers. Most cases of HL arise from preapoptotic germinal center B cells that cannot synthesize immunoglobulin. The R-S cell appears to be resistant to apoptotic stimuli. Deregulation of the nuclear transcription factor nuclear factor kappa B (NFkB) in the R-S cells may explain this resistance to apoptosis [21, 22].

Other characteristic terms that are useful in the diagnosis of HL include "Hodgkin cell" may be used for mononuclear variants. "Mummified cells" are neoplastic cells that contain condensed cytoplasm and pyknotic reddish nuclei. "Lacunar cells" have multilobated nuclei, small nucleoli, and abundant, pale cytoplasm that often "retracts" during tissue fixation and sectioning, leaving the nucleus in what appears to be an empty space (lacune). The "lymphocytic and histiocytic" (LandH) variants, sometimes referred to as "popcorn cells" have vesicular, polylobulated nuclei and distinct, small, usually peripheral nucleoli, without perinucleolar halos.

Histology

The WHO classifies HL into classical HL and nodular lymphocyte predominant HL. A revised European-American Classification of Lymphoid Neoplasms (REAL classification), has been proposed.

The REAL/WHO classification differs from older classifications in several ways. In the REAL classification, HL is subdivided into lymphocytic predominance, nodular (with or without diffuse areas), and the other forms of classical HL: nodular sclerosis, mixed cellularity, lymphocyte-depletion types and lymphocyte-rich classic disease [23-25].

Table 1. Immunophenotypic Markers in HL

Class of HL	CD15	CD19	CD20	CD22	CD30	CD45	CD79
Classical	++	-		+	++	-	-
NLPHL	-	++	++	++	+/-	-	++

+ = 20-30% expression; ++ = >70% expression.

"Classical" HL, which includes the nodular sclerosis Hodgkin lymphoma (NSHL), mixed cellularity HL (MCHL), lymphocyte rich classical HL (LRCHL), and lymphocyte depleted (LDHL) subtypes.

Nodular lymphocyte predominant HL (NLPHL) is in class by itself.

IMMUNOPHENOTYPE

Tumor cells in classic HL do not express B cell antigens such as CD45, CD19 and CD79a, but virtually all express CD30. In classical HL, the RS cells typically express CD15 (85 percent of cases) and CD30 and usually lack global expression of pan-B (CD19, CD20, CD79a) and pan-T (CD3, CD7) antigen [26]; however, many cases of classical HL have B cell antigen expression of CD20 on R-S cells [27, 28]. Among classical forms of HL, CD20 expression is most frequently seen in the lymphocyte-rich HL subtype [29-31].

In comparison, the tumor cells of HLPHL do express B cell antigens such as CD19, CD20, CD22 and CD79 [32-33]. Table 1 shows the common immunophenotypic markers in HL.

CLINICAL PRESENTATION

Eighty percent of patients present with painless adenopathy, most commonly in the supraclavicular or cervical area. The involved lymph node is usually nontender with a rubbery consistency. The most common involved site is in the neck. Enlarged nodes are found in the axilla in 10 to 20 percent of patients and inguinal nodes are involved in 6 to 12 percent [34-36].

Although not detectable on physical examination, the mediastinal nodes are involved in 60 to 70 percent of cases at presentation, and retroperitoneal nodes in 25 percent. Exclusive infradiaphragmatic lymphadenopathy is infrequent, occurring in less than 10 percent of individuals. Adolescents and young adults present with a mediastinal mass 75% of the time. Children less than 10 years of age present with mediastinal disease only 35% of the time; this is thought to be due to these patients having either mixed cellularity or lymphocyte predominant histology. Less commonly, the mass produces nonspecific symptoms such as retrosternal chest pain, cough, or shortness of breath. Small pericardial or pleural effusions are rare except in patients with bulky mediastinal disease. Superior vena caval obstruction is also rare.

Approximately 20% of patients will have *bulky adenopathy*, which can be defined as, a large mediastinal mass with a maximum diameter that is greater than one third of the chest diameter and/or a node or nodal aggregate greater than 10 centimeters [36]. The definition of bulk disease can differ from one study to the next. 80 to 85% of children and adolescents will also have involvement of lymph nodes/and or spleen only (stages I-III). 15 to 20% of patients will have noncontiguous extranodal involvement (stage IV); with the most common sites of extranodal involvement being the lung, bone marrow, bone and liver.

A significant proportion of patients with Hodgkin lymphoma develop systemic symptoms prior to the discovery of lymphadenopathy. Typical constitutional symptoms, called B symptoms, include fever (>100.4), night sweats (presence of drenching night sweats), and unexplained weight loss greater than 10% of body weight over the past six months.

Other symptoms that may be present are pruritis. Although not defined as a B symptom, pruritus may be an important early symptom, preceding the diagnosis of Hodgkin lymphoma by months or even a year or more [36]. Pruritus occurs early in approximately 10 to 15 percent of patients, but the great majority of patients experience pruritus at some time during the course of illness. It is usually generalized and occasionally severe enough to cause intense scratching and excoriations. Severe, but not mild, pruritus is a poor prognostic sign [36].

More rarely, patients with HL can have severe pain following alcohol ingestion [37], skin lesions [38, 39], and hypercalcemia, which may be due to bony involvement or more often to increased production of calcitriol (1,25-dihydroxyvitamin D3) [40, 41]. Hematological manifestations can include: anemia, which can be normochromic and normocytic or, rarely, a Coombs' positive hemolytic anemia that may be associated with immune thrombocytopenia [42, 43], eosinophilia (due to production of chemokines, such as interleukin-5 and eotaxin, that stimulate eosinophil production and/or recruitment) [44, 45], Leukocytosis, thrombocytosis, and lymphopenia, are also seen with Hodgkin lymphoma, especially in patients with advanced stage disease.

Some uncommon presenting symptoms include chest pain, bronchial obstruction, abdominal pain, bone pain, spinal cord compression, and peripheral edema.

Patterns of Disease Presentation

Hodgkin lymphoma spreads via the lymph nodes. It is widely accepted that Hodgkin lymphoma starts at a single site within the lymphatic system, usually a lymph node, and then progresses to adjacent lymph nodes via lymphatic channels before disseminating to distant nonadjacent sites and organs [46]. Noncontiguous spread and hematologic distribution are more common with recurrent disease.

Diagnostic Evaluation and Staging

The diagnostic workup for HL includes a detailed history and a thorough physical examination. Staging is based on a combination of physical and imaging studies. Staging and evaluation of disease status is done initially at the diagnosis and performed again early in the course of treatment and at the end of treatment.

It is important for the diagnostic workup to begin with a detailed history of signs and B symptoms and a physical examination that documents the sites and size of all adenopathy as well as splenic involvement and organ dysfunction.

Computed tomography (CT) scans of the neck, thorax, abdomen and pelvis should be performed to help determine the status of intrathoracic lymph node groups (including hila and cardophrenic angle), lung parenchyma, pericardium, pleura and the chest wall. In addition, an upright chest radiograph (CXR) should be performed with posteroanterior (PA) and lateral views to document any mediastinal disease [47, 48]. The CXR is important for establishing the criterion of bulky mediastinal lymphadenopathy.

Along with CT, nuclear imaging is important for staging HL and for monitoring response to therapy. Functional imaging such as fluorodeoxyglucose positron emission tomography (FDG-PET) is a reliable method to assess bone involvement and may be useful in demonstrating unsuspected lesions in the spleen. FDG-PET has been recommended as the functional imaging procedure for initial staging. FDG-PET has advantages over traditional gallium-67 scintography as it is a one day procedure with higher resolution, better dosimetry and less intestinal activity [49-52]. In addition, with newer imaging techniques and equipment, combined CT-PET scans can evaluate disease simultaneously with both modalities. Technetium-99 bone scintography should be performed in patients with bone pain or elevated alkaline phosphatase.

Laboratory studies include a complete blood count, chemistries to evaluate liver and renal function and acute phase reactants such as ferritin, and erythrocyte sedimentation rate, which may be seen as nonspecific markers of tumor activity.

Biopsy

Surgical procedures for staging and diagnosis of HL include bone marrow biopsies and lymph node biopsies though care needs to be taken when administering anesthesia. Patients with large mediastinal masses are at risk for cardiac or respiratory compromise during anesthesia or sedation. Bilateral bone marrow biopsies are recommended for patients with B symptoms or those with higher stage (Stage III or IV). After a careful and thorough physical examination and imaging has been undertaken, the least invasive procedure should be used to establish the diagnosis of lymphoma. If possible, the diagnosis should be established by lymph node biopsy. Fine needle biopsy is not recommended because of the small number of cells present in the specimen may be inadequate for immunophenotyping needed to classify HL into one of the subtypes.

Staging

After a diagnosis of HL is made, the clinical stage of disease is determined to guide treatment and act as a measure of prognosis. The main goals of staging are to measure the extent of disease and associated prognostic factors, and to define disease manifestations that can be reevaluated during and after treatment to determine the effectiveness of therapy. Staging also serves an important role for the comparison of treatments among studies.

The staging classification currently used for HL is the Ann Arbor Classification and is found in Table 2. The Ann Arbor Classification was originally adopted in 1971 and was updated in 1989 [53, 54]. In 1988, the Cotswold modifications added valuable information regarding the presence of bulky disease and the efficacy of imaging studies for staging [55].

Table 2. Modified Ann Arbor Classification of Hodgkin Lymphoma

A. Stage	Description
I:	Involvement of single lymph node region (I) or localized involvement of a single extralymphatic organ or site (E)
II:	Involvement of two or more lymph node regions on the same side of the diaphragm (II) or localized contiguous involvement or a single extralymphatic organ or site and its regional lymph node(s) with involvement of one or more lymph node regions on the same side of the diaphragm (IIE)
III:	Involvement of lymph node regions on both sides of the diaphragm (III), which may also be accompanied by localized contiguous involvement of an extralymphatic organ or site (IIIE), by involvement of the spleen (IIIS), or both (IIIS+E)
IV:	Disseminated (multifocal) involvement of one or more extralymphatic organs or tissue, with or without associated lymph node involvement, or isolated extralymphatic organ involvement with distant (nonregional) nodal involvement
B:	Symptoms and Presentation
A symptoms:	Lack of "B" symptoms
B symptoms:	At least one of the following: Unexplained weight loss > 10% in the preceding 6 months Unexplained recurrent fever > 38°C Drenching night sweats
X:	Bulky disease: > 10 cm in maximum dimension or involves > 1/3 of the chest diameter (seen on chest x-ray)
S:	Splenic involvement
E:	Involvement of a single extranodal site that is contiguous or proximal to the known nodal site

Lister TA, Crowther D, Sutcliffe SB et al.: Report of a committee convened to discuss the evaluation and staging of patients with Hodgkin's disease: Cotswalds meeting. J Clin Oncol 7 (11): 1630-6, 1989.

All cases of HL are subclassified to indicate the absence (A) or presence (B) of "B" symptoms. "B" symptoms are defined as one or more of the following three systemic symptoms: significant unexplained fever, night sweats, or unexplained weight loss exceeding 10 percent of body weight during the six months prior to diagnosis.

The subscript "X" is used if bulky disease is present. No subscripts are used in the absence of bulk.

The subscript "S" is used if the spleen is involved with HL. Splenic involvement is noted when there are multiple focal defects, that are neither cystic nor vascular, noted on at least two imaging techniques. Two independent scans (ie, both PET and CT) are needed to determine disease involvement because of the high false positivity of the PET scan alone.

The subscript "E" is used if limited extranodal extension is documented. More extensive extranodal disease is designated stage IV.

Patients with stage I or stage II disease are then further stratified for treatment purposes into favorable and unfavorable prognosis disease based upon the presence or absence of certain clinical features, such as age, B symptoms, and large mediastinaladenopathy.

Table 3. Clinical Staging System

Early Favorable

- Clinical Stage I or II without any risk factors

Early Unfavorable

- Clinical stage I or II with one or more of the following risk factors:
    - Large mediastinal mass (>33% of the thoracic width on the chest x-ray, ≥10 cm on CT scan).
    - Extranodal involvement.
    - Elevated erythrocyte sedimentation rate (>30 mm/h for B stage, >50 mm/h for A stage).
    - Three or more lymph node areas' involvement.
    - B symptoms.

Advanced Favorable

- Clinical stage III or IV with zero to three adverse risk factors listed below [58].
    - Albumin level of <4.0 g/dL.
    - Hemoglobin level of <10.5 g/dL.
    - Male sex.
    - Age of ≥45 years.
    - Stage IV disease.
    - White blood cell (WBC) count of ≥15,000/mm^3.
    - Absolute lymphocytic count of <600/mm^3 or a lymphocyte count that was <8% of the total WBC count.

Advanced Unfavorable

- Clinical stage III or IV with four or more adverse risk factors listed above [58].

Many investigators and many new clinical trials employ a clinical staging system that divides patients into four major groups early favorable, early unfavorable, advanced favorable and advanced unfavorable [56, 57]. The criteria for these four groups are listed in Table 3.

Prognostic Factors

Several pretreatment factors have been associated with an adverse outcome in one or more studies and these include: advanced stage of disease, the presence of B symptoms, and the presence of bulk disease, extranodal extension, male sex, and elevated erythrocyte sedimentation rate.

Histology has been noted to be an important prognostic indicator as well. Patients with NLPHL appear to have an overall better prognosis than those with CHL [59]. Serum markers are currently being studied as prognostic indicators; those associated with poor prognosis include: tumor necrosis factor, soluble CD30, beta 2 macrogloblin, transferring, and serum IL-10 level [59-63]. Favorable outcomes have been noted with high levels of capase 3 in Reed Sternberg cells [64].

Other prognostic indicators include initial response to chemotherapy. Early response assessment is based on volume reduction of disease, functional imaging status or both [65-67]. Studies have shown that adult individuals with advanced favorable disease have a 60% to 80% freedom-from-progression at 5 years from treatment with first-line chemotherapy [58]; while those with advanced unfavorable disease showed a 42% to 51% freedom-from-progression at 5 years from treatment with first-line chemotherapy [58].

In children and adolescents prognostic factors include staging, gender, along with disease staging. Studies done by Stanford-St.Jude-Dana Farber Cancer Institute consortium noted that in children with clinically staged HL, male gender, stage IIB, IIIB, or IV disease; white blood cell count 11,500/mm^3 or higher; and hemogblobin less than 11.0 g/dl were prognostic factors associated with inferior disease free survival and overall survival [68]. In the CCG-5942 study, the combination of B symptoms and bulky diease was noted to be inferior prognostic indicators [69].

Significant reduction in disease volume and PET negativity after 2 cycles of chemotherapy is associated with a favorable outcome in children and adolescents [70, 71]. This therapeutic response allows investigators and clinicians to reduce chemotherapy and radiation for individuals and is being studied in cooperative groups.

Treatment

Treatment Overview

In general, the use of combined chemotherapy and low dose involved field radiation therapy (IFRT) allows for maximal therapy with reduction of individual drug related or radiation related toxicities. The volume of radiation and the intensity/duration of chemotherapy is determined by prognostic factors at presentation and include the presence of B symptoms, initial stage of disease and presence of bulky disease. Due to the large number of severe long term effects presented with HL therapy, cooperative groups have tailored HL therapy for young children to include reduction of alkylating agents, anthyracyline agents and radiation dose and volume. Adults generally receive combination chemotherapy as initial treatment based on prognostic factors. Adult patients with nonbulky stage IA or IIA disease are considered to have clinical early-stage disease and are candidates for chemotherapy, combined modality therapy, or radiation therapy alone. When chemotherapy alone or combined modality therapy is applied, laparotomy is not required. Adults with higher stages, Stage III or IV will require combination chemotherapy with or without additional radiation therapy. A summary of common protocols and chemotherapy is found in table 4.

Radiation is an important component of HL therapy; though the doses are modificed in pediatric or advanced stage patients. Historically, radiation was used as monotherapy in Stage I or II HL adult patients; however, contemporary therapy uses combined chemotherapy and radiotherapy. In adult HL, the appropriate dose of radiation alone is 25 Gy to 30 Gy to clinically uninvolved sites and 35 Gyto 44 Gy to regions of initial nodal involvement [72-75]. Radiation is usually given to the neck, chest, and axilla (mantle field) and then to an abdominal field to treat para-aortic nodes and the spleen (splenic pedicle). In some patients, pelvic nodes are treated with a third field. The three fields constitute total nodal radiation therapy. In some cases, the pelvic and para-aortic nodes are treated in a single field called an inverted Y. In patients with lower stage therapy and favorable histology, treatment of the pelvic lymph nodes is frequently omitted, since fertility can be preserved without affecting relapse-free survival. Guidelines for radiation are listed in table 5.

Table 4. Common chemotherapy protocols

Acronym	Chemotherapy agents
ABV	Doxorubicin, bleomycin, vinblastine
ABVD	Doxorubicin, bleomycin, vinblastine, dacarbazine (DITC)
BEACOPP	Bleomycin, etoposide, doxorubicin, cyclophosphamide, vincristine, procarnazine, prednisone
CHOP	Cyclophosphamide, doxorubicin, vincristine, prednisone
COP(P)	Cyclophosphamide, vincristine, procarbazine, (prednisone)
D(A)ABVE(PC)	Doxorubicin, bleomycin, vincristine, etoposide, (prednisone, cyclphosphamide)
MOPP	Mechlorethamine (nitrogen mustard), vincristine, procarbazine, prednisone
VAMP	Vincristine, doxorubicin, methotrexate, prednisone
VEPA	Vinblastine, etoposide, prednisone, doxorubicin
OEPA	Vincristine, etoposide, prednisone, doxorubicin
OPPA	Vincristine, procarbazine, prednisone, doxorubicin
ICE	Ifosphamide, carboplatin, etoposide
IV	Ifosphamide, vinorelabine
R-ICE	Rituximab, ifosphamide, carboplatin, etoposide
BEAM	Carmustine, etoposide, cytarabine, melphalan

Table 5. Guidelines for involved field radiation

Involved nodes	Radiation therapy field
Cervical	Neck, supraclavicular/infraclavicular
Supraclavicular	Neck and infraclavicular/supraclavicular,±axilla
Axilla	Axilla ± infraclavicular/supraclavicular
Mediastinum	Mediastinum, hila, infraclavicular/supraclavicular
Hila	Hila, mediastinum
Spleen	Spleen ± para-aortics
Para-aortics	Para-aortics ± spleen
Iliac	Ipsilateraliliacs, inguinal + femoral
Inguinal	Inguinal + femoral ± iliac
Femoral	Inguinal + femoral ± iliac

Volume considerations for treatment are often protocol specific but generally include the initial involved lymph node regions. Additional considerations relate to the location of the disease (pericardium and chest wall). Ideally the ovaries should be exposed to less than 3Gy to preserve fertility. The testes may be exposed to 5-10% of the administered pelvic dose; this low dose can cause azoopsermia depending on the total pelvic dose. It is important to restrict radiation therapy to areas of bulky disease while still protecting normal tissue. This can often be accomplished by careful positioning of the patient and by customizing shield blocks. Large volume radiation therapy can compromise organ function and may limit the intensity of retrieval therapy if relapse occurs.

Treatment for Early Favorable Histology Individuals

Patients are designated as having early favorable Hodgkin lymphoma (HL) if they have clinical stage I or stage II disease and no adverse risk factors which include B symptoms, extranodal disease, bulky disease, three or more sites of nodal involvement or a sedimentation rate ≥50 mm/h. Historically, patients with stage I or II disease received monotherapy with radiation; however studies done in the 1990's with patient with favorable prognostic Hodgkin (H8-F) and unfavorable prognostic Hodgkin (H8-U) showed that patients who received combination chemotherapy with MOPP-ABV plus involved field radiation had 5 year event free survival that was close to 98% versus 74% for those that received radiation alone [76]. A randomized prospective trial from the National Cancer Institute of Canada involving 123 patients with early favorable HL compared ABVD for four to six cycles to subtotal nodal radiation; with a median follow-up of 4.2 years, no difference was observed in event-free survival (88% vs. 87%; *P* = .60) or in overall survival (OS) (97% vs. 100%; *P* = .30) [77]. Recent trials have focused on decreasing the amount of chemotherapy and radiation to help decrease the late effects that are known to occur post Hodgkin therapy.

Treatment for Early Unfavorable Histology Individuals

Early unfavorable HL individuals are those whohave clinical stage I or stage II disease and one or more of the following risk factors: B symptoms (fever ≥38°C, soaking night sweats, weight loss ≥10% within 6 months), extranodal disease, bulky disease (≥10 cm or >33% of the chest diameter on chest x-ray), three or more sites of nodal involvement or sedimentation rate of ≥50 mm/h. Historically, patients with early unfavorable HL had a poor prognosis with radiation alone; with EFS of 30% at 5 years [78]. The current standard of care uses ABVD for 4-6 cycles plus involved field radiation. Current studies have shown that the number of cycles of chemotherapy do increase the EFS at 5 years, though increased therapy does have increased toxicity [79-81].

Treatment for Advanced Favorable Histology Individuals

Patients with clinical stage III or IV with less than three adverse factors are clinically staged as advanced favorable histology individuals. For over two decades, the standard of care for those with advanced favorable histology was using the MOPP regimen. However, the MOPP regimen had long term toxicities that included secondary myelodysplastic syndromes, leukemias and infertility in both males and females. When MOPP therapy was compared to ABVD in 361 patients; ABVD therapy for 6 to 8 months was shown to be as effective as 12 months of MOPP alternating with ABVD, and both were superior to MOPP alone in terms of failure-free survival (FFS) (50% vs. 36% with a 14-year median follow-up [82-83].

Other regimens that were compared to the ABVD were BECOPP and CEC; in a prospective randomized trial of 307 patients with advanced-stage disease, including IIB disease and advanced-favorable Hodgkin lymphoma patients, compared ABVD, BEACOPP (four escalated courses plus two standard courses), and CEC.[84] With a median follow-up of

41 months, although progression-free survival favored BEACOPP over ABVD (78% vs. 68%, $P = .038$), there was no significant difference in OS [84].

Treatment for Advanced Unfavorable Histology Individuals

Unfortunately, treatment strategies are not as standardized for patients with advanced unfavorable histology. Many regimens have been used including, ABVD, BEACOPP, and COPP/ABVD. The German Hodgkin Lymphoma Study Group (HD9 trial) randomly assigned 1,201 patients with advanced-stage disease to COPP/ABVD, BEACOPP, or to increased-dose BEACOPP, with most patients receiving consolidative radiation therapy to sites of initial bulky disease (≥5 cm) [85]. The 10-year OS rates from time of treatment were 75% for COPP/ABVD, 80% for BEACOPP, and 86% for increased-dose BEACOPP. Clinical trials are addressing the role of more intensive regimens for patients with advanced-stage disease and poor prognostic factors. Controversy exists about whether the optimal strategy should involve early dose intensification, with subsequent risks of increased late toxic effects (such as leukemia) or whether ABVD should be employed and patients who relapse be salvaged with high-dose treatment and autografting. In a prospective randomized trial of 163 patients with unfavorable advanced-stage disease who attained a complete or partial remission after four cycles of ABVD, no difference was observed in OS or FFS either with high-dose therapy with autologous stem cell transplant or with four more cycles of ABVD [86].

Treatment for Children and Adolescents

Due to the large number of severe long term effects presented with HL therapy, cooperative groups have tailored HL therapy for young children to include reduction of alkylating agents, anthyracyline agents and radiation dose and volume. Pediatric oncologists agree that standard dose radiation therapy; particularly applied to large volumes including critical organs normally in the mantle field have unacceptable toxicities which include growth dysfunction, increased risk for breast cancer in young females and cardiovascular complications [87-88]. Thus, all children and adolescents generally receive combination chemotherapy as initial treatment based on prognostic factors. The general treatment strategy for children with HL is to use chemotherapy for all patients with or without radiation. The number of cycles and intensity of chemotherapy may be determined by rapidity and degree of response, as is the radiation dose and volume.

Between 1987 and 2001, the Children's Cancer Group (CCG), the Pediatric Oncology Group (POG) and the Dana Farber-Stanford-St. Jude Pediatric Hodgkin's Consortium (PHC) and the German pediatric cooperative groups (DAL and GPOH) have conducted the largest risk adapted therapeutic studies for children and adolescents with HL. ABVD was developed by POG, when it was noted that regimens such as MOPP [89] containing alkylating agents were shown to be an increased risk for chemotherapy induced leukemia.

CCG and POG have attempted to decrease or eliminate radiation therapy in HL patients. In the CCG 521 study, patients were randomized between 12 cycles of alternating MOPP/ABVD and 6 cycles of ABVD plus low dose regional chemotherapy; EFS was lower at 77% for Stage III and Stage IV patients [90]. CCG 5942 studied the elimination of radiation therapy in a randomized fashion in all patients who had complete response following chemotherapy. Patients were treated with different numbers of cycles of COPP/ABV, cytarabine, etoposide and CHOP depending on their initial stage and bulk of disease. Eighty-three percent of patients were noted to have complete response and 60% were randomized to receive either IFRT or no further therapy. Event free survival at 4 years was over 80% for stage II and IV patients. Overall EFS was 91% for the group who received IFRT and 86% for those who did not [91].

Current COG studies (representing a merger of CCG and POG) continue to focus on decreasing long term effects by minimizing radiation and chemotherapy. Most recently, COG has studies open for low risk HL (AHOD0431) and intermediate risk HL (AHOD0031). AHOD0431 is evaluating patients with stage I or IIA with no bulk disease using 3 cycles of AVPC. These patients do not receive any etoposide or bleomycin. Those patients who receive a complete remission after three cycles of chemotherapy do not receive any further treatment. Patients who achieve partial remission after three cycles receive LD-IFRT. The COG Intermediate risk trial, AHOD0031 is evaluating early response after 2 cycles of ABVE-PC to determine subsequent therapy in stages I and II with either B symptoms or bulk disease, stage IIAE, stage IIIA and stage IVA. Response is based on imaging with PET scan and CT scans.

Treatment for NLPHL

Nodular lymphocyte–predominant HL is a clinicopathologic entity of B-cell origin that is distinct from classic HL [92, 93]. Patients with lymphocyte-predominant disease have earlier-stage disease, longer survival, and fewer treatment failures than those with classic HL [94]. Despite a usually favorable prognosis, there is a tendency for histologic transformation to diffuse large B-cell lymphoma in around 10% of patients by 10 years [95]. Lymphocyte-predominant HL is usually diagnosed in asymptomatic young males with cervical or inguinal lymph nodes but usually without mediastinal involvement. Based on retrospective analyses spanning several decades and because of the rarity of this histology, limited-field radiation therapy is the most common treatment approach for patients with early-stage disease [96-98]. Recent studies have shown that a systemic therapy with MOPP combined with monoclonal antibody therapy may be beneficial [99].

Treatment for Relapsed

Relapsed patients can still be cured even if relapse occurs after initial treatment. Relapse usually occurs within the first four years following treatment. The presence of B symptoms and extranodal disease at the time of relapse are poor prognostic features. Currently there is no standard reinduction protocol for HL though there are a spectrum of treatment options that exist. Potentially curative options include conventional chemotherapy/radiation therapy protocols for those with low risk relapses, radiation therapy alone for those relapsing in a limited nodal pattern and reinduction chemotherapy followed by autologouos hematopoietic stem cell transplantation for those with more advanced stages. Combination chemotherapy regimens are listed in table 6. Autologous stem cells are used because there is an increased risk of mortality associated with allogeneic stem cells. Following autologous stem cell transplant, the projected survival rate is 45% to 70% and progression free survival is 30% to 65% [100]. For those patients who fail autologous stem cell transplant or for patients who cannot mobilize sufficient numbers of autologous stem cells, allogeneic stem cells have been used with varying degrees of success. LD-IFRT to sites of relapsed disease should be given even if these sites had not received previous radiation. LD-IFRT is usually administered after high dose chemotherapy and stem cell rescue. Patients treated with stem cell transplant may experience relapse as late as 5 years after their transplant; they should be monitored closely for relapse along with long term effects.

Patients with progressive or primary refractory HL have poor salvage rates even with stem cell transplant and radiation therapy.

Table 6. Combination regimens used in the treatment of Relapsed/Recurrent Hodgkin Disease

Acronym	Chemotherapy Agents
ICE	Ifosphamide, carboplatin, etoposide
DECAL	Dexamethasone, etoposide, cisplatin, cytarabine, and L-asparaginase
DECA	Dexamethasone, etoposide, cisplatin, cytarabine
IV	Ifosphamide and vinorelbine
GV	Gemcitabine and vinorelbine
IEP-ABVD-COPP	Ifosphamide, etoposide, prednisone-doxorubicin, bleomycin, vinblastine, dacarbazine-cyclophosphamide, vincristine, procarbazine, prednisone
APE	Cytosine, arabinoside, cisplatin, etoposide
BEAM *	Carmustine (BCNU), etoposide, cytarabine, melphalan
Other transplant regimens include:	Thiotepa, etoposide combined with either cyclophosphamide, carboplatin or melphalan

* Most commonly used preparative regimen for peripheral blood stem cell transplant.

Long Term Complications

Survivors of HL are at risk for numerous late complications of chemotherapy and radiation therapy. Late effects include secondary malignancies, organ dysfunction, and psychosocial sequelae. The late effects of therapy are worse in children and adolescent survivors of HL.

Secondary Malignancies

A number of large studies have evaluated the incidence of malignancies in survivors of childhood and adolescent survivors [91, 101-105] and have reported between a 7 to 18 times higher risk of secondary malignancies when compared to the general population. Many of the patients included in these large cohorts received high dose alkylating agents and radiation doses. Secondary hematological malignancies in HL survivors (most commonly acute myeloid leukemias and myeloid dysplasia) are related to the use of alkylating agents, anthracycline and etoposide. The risk of leukemia appears to plateau at 10-15 years post therapy while the risk of second solid malignancies increases [101, 105, 106]. Female survivors of HL have an increased risk for breast cancer that is directly related to the dose of radiation therapy received. There is a 3.2 fold increase in the risk of developing breast cancer for females who received 4 Gy and an eight fold increase in risk for females who received 40 Gy [101, 107,108]. Female patients treated with both radiation therapy and alkylating agent chemotherapy have a lower relative risk of developing breast cancer than women who received radiation therapy alone [109]. Second solid tumors in patients receiving radiation of at least 35 Gy are consistently noted.

Cardiac Toxicity

HL survivors exposed to doxorubicin or thoracic radiation therapy are at an increased risk for long term toxicity. The risks to the heart are related to cumulative anthracycline dose, metehod of administration, amount of radiation delivered to different depths of the heart, volume and specific areas of the heart irradiated, total and fractional irradiation doses, age at exposure, latency periods and gender. Late effects to the heart include: delayed pericarditis, pancarditis (which includes pericardial and myocardial fibrosis), myopathy, coronary artery disease, functional valve injury and conduction injuries. Nontherapeutic risk factors for coronary heart disease including family history, obesity, smoking, hypertension, diabetes and hypercholesterolemia are likely to impact the frequency of disease. Increased risk of doxorubicin related cardiomyopathy is associated with female sex, cumulative doses higher than 200 mg/m2 to 300 mg/m2, younger age at time of exposure and increased time from exposure [110-120].

Pulmonary Dysfunction

Pulmonary fibrosis is a late complication of HL following radiation therapy. Bleomycin associated pulmonary fibrosis with decreased diffusion capacity is most commonly seen following doses greater than 200-400 units/m2 [121-123]. Acute pneumonitis as evidenced by fever, congestion, cough and dyspnea can follow radiation therapy along at doses greater than 40 Gy to focal lung volumes or after lower doses (15-20 Gy) when combined with chemotherapy and including generous or whole lung volumes.

Thyroid Dysfunction

Primary hypothyroidism is the most common thyroid dysfunction noted following radiation therapy to the neck for HL; though hyperthyroidism, goiter or nodules have also been noted. The incidence of thyroid dysfunction varies with the dose of radiation and the length of follow-up. For hypothyroidism, there is a clear dose response with a 20 year risk of 20 percent for those with had received less than 35 Gy, 30 percent following 35-44.9 Gy and 50 percent following greater than 45 Gy to the thyroid gland [124]. The risk for both hypo and hyper thyroidism increases in the first 3-5 years after diagnosis. The incidence of nodules increased 10 years from the time of diagnosis [125].

Gonadal Dysfunction and Infertility

Male Gonadal Toxicity

Gonadal toxicity in males is likely to manifest as infertility, lack of sexual development, small atrophic testicles, and sexual dysfunction. Infertility caused by azzospermia is the most common manifestation of gonadal toxicity. Alkylating agents and radiation therapy are common agents associated with male infertility. Males who receive less than 4 gm/m2 of cyclophosphamide without testicular radiation or any other alkylating agents are likely to retain their fertility. Cumulative doses of cyclophosphamide greater than 9 gm/m2 are likely to result in infertility [126, 127]. Radiation doses less than 30 Gy are unlikely to affect endocrine function and boys usually progress through puberty normally [128]. There can be temporary oligospermia following low doses of radiation though permanent azoospermia.

Female Gonadal Toxicity

The risk of female gonadal toxicity increased with age at treatment. Menstrual irregularities including amenorrhea and premature ovarian failure occur more commonly in women treated with cyclophosphamide and other alkylating agents than in adolescent and prepubertal females. Several studies have shown that the incidence of early menopause in young female survivors of HL may be as high as 37% [129, 130].

Monitoring for Adverse Long Term Outcomes

Specific long-term follow-up guidelines after treatment of childhood cancer have been published by the Children's Oncology Group, and are available at www. survivorshipguidelines.org. To date, there are not uniformly effective long term follow-up plans for survivors of adult HL.

REFERENCES

[1] Jemal A, Siegel R, Ward E, et al. Cancer statistics, 2009. CA *Cancer J. Clin.* 2009; 59:225.

[2] Ries LA, Kosary CL, Hankey BF, et al. (Eds). SEER cancer statistics review: 1973-1994, NIH publ no. 97-2789, National Cancer Institute, Bethesda 1997.

[3] Correa P, O'Conor GT. Epidemiologic patterns of Hodgkin's disease. *Int. J. Cancer* 1971; 8:192.

[4] Correa P, O'Conor GT. Geographic pathology of lymphoreticular tumors: summary of survey from the geographic pathology committee of the international union against cancer. *J. Natl. Cancer Inst.* 1973; 50:1609.

[5] Gutensohn N, Cole P. Childhood social environment and Hodgkin's disease. *N. Engl. J. Med.* 1981; 304:135.

[6] Devesa, S.S., et al., Recent cancer trends in the United States. *J. Natl. Cancer Inst.*, 1995. 87(3): p. 175-82.

[7] Kersey, J.H., R.S. Shapiro, and A.H. Filipovich, Relationship of immunodeficiency to lymphoid malignancy. *Pediatr. Infect. Dis. J.*, 1988. 7(5 Suppl): p. S10-2.

[8] Mack, T.M., et al., Concordance for Hodgkin's disease in identical twins suggesting genetic susceptibility to the young-adult form of the disease. *N. Engl. J. Med.*, 1995. 332(7): p. 413-8.

[9] Stiller, C.A., What causes Hodgkin's disease in children? *Eur. J. Cancer*, 1998. 34(4): p. 523-8.

[10] Grufferman, S. and E. Delzell, Epidemiology of Hodgkin's disease. *Epidemiol. Rev.*, 1984. 6: p. 76-106.

[11] McNally RJ, Alston RD, Cairns DP, et al. Geographical and ecological analyses of childhood acute leukaemias and lymphomas in north-west England. *Br. J. Haematol.* 2003; 123:60.

[12] Hu E, Hufford S, Lukes R, et al. Third-World Hodgkin's disease at Los Angeles County-University of Southern California Medical Center. *J. Clin. Oncol.* 1988; 6:1285.

[13] Goedert JJ, Coté TR, Virgo P, et al. Spectrum of AIDS-associated malignant disorders. *Lancet* 1998; 351:1833.
[14] Tinguely M, Vonlanthen R, Müller E, et al. Hodgkin's disease-like lymphoproliferative disorders in patients with different underlying immunodeficiency states. *Mod. Pathol.* 1998; 11:307.
[15] Glaser SL, Clarke CA, Gulley ML, et al. Population-based patterns of human immunodeficiency virus-related Hodgkin lymphoma in the Greater San Francisco Bay Area, 1988-1998. *Cancer* 2003; 98:300.
[16] Garnier JL, Lebranchu Y, Dantal J, et al. Hodgkin's disease after transplantation. *Transplantation* 1996; 61:71.
[17] Patel P, Hanson DL, Sullivan PS, et al. Incidence of types of cancer among HIV-infected persons compared with the general population in the United States, 1992-2003. *Ann. Intern. Med.* 2008; 148:728.
[18] Brauninger, A., et al., Molecular biology of Hodgkin's and Reed/Sternberg cells in Hodgkin's lymphoma. *Int. J. Cancer*, 2006. 118(8): p. 1853-61.
[19] Staudt, L.M., The molecular and cellular origins of Hodgkin's disease. *J. Exp. Med.*, 2000. 191(2): p. 207-12.
[20] Kuppers, R., et al., Biology of Hodgkin's lymphoma. *Ann. Oncol.*, 2002. 13 Suppl 1: p. 11-8.
[21] Baeuerle, P.A. and D. Baltimore, NF-kappa B: ten years after. *Cell*, 1996. 87(1): p. 13-20.
[22] Karin, M. and M. Delhase, The I kappa B kinase (IKK) and NF-kappa B: key elements of proinflammatory signalling. *Semin. Immunol.*, 2000. 12(1): p. 85-98.
[23] Harris, N.L., Hodgkin's lymphomas: classification, diagnosis, and grading. *Semin. Hematol.*, 1999. 36(3): p. 220-32.
[24] Pileri, S.A., et al., Hodgkin's lymphoma: the pathologist's viewpoint. *J. Clin. Pathol.*, 2002. 55(3): p. 162-76.
[25] Pileri, S.A., et al., Primary follicular lymphoma of the testis in childhood: an entity with peculiar clinical and molecular characteristics. *J. Clin. Pathol.*, 2002. 55(9): p. 684-8.
[26] vonWasielewski R, Mengel M, Fischer R, et al. Classical Hodgkin's disease. Clinical impact of the immunophenotype. *Am. J. Pathol.* 1997; 151:1123.
[27] Zukerberg LR, Collins AB, Ferry JA, Harris NL. Coexpression of CD15 and CD20 by Reed-Sternberg cells in Hodgkin's disease. *Am. J. Pathol.* 1991; 139:475.
[28] Schmid C, Pan L, Diss T, Isaacson PG. Expression of B-cell antigens by Hodgkin's and Reed-Sternberg cells. *Am. J. Pathol.* 1991; 139:701.
[29] vonWasielewski R, Werner M, Fischer R, et al. Lymphocyte-predominant Hodgkin's disease. An immunohistochemical analysis of 208 reviewed Hodgkin's disease cases from the German Hodgkin Study Group. *Am. J. Pathol.* 1997; 150:793.
[30] Sextro M, Diehl V, Franklin J, et al. Lymphocyte predominant Hodgkin's disease--a workshop report. European Task Force on Lymphoma. *Ann. Oncol.* 1996; 7 Suppl 4:61.
[31] Ashton-Key M, Thorpe PA, Allen JP, Isaacson PG. Follicular Hodgkin's disease. *Am. J. Surg. Pathol.* 1995; 19:1294.
[32] Skinnider, B.F. and T.W. Mak, The role of cytokines in classical Hodgkin lymphoma. *Blood*, 2002. 99(12): p. 4283-97.
[33] Tzankov, A., et al., Expression of B-cell markers in classical hodgkin lymphoma: a tissue microarray analysis of 330 cases. *Mod. Pathol.*, 2003. 16(11): p. 1141-7.

[34] Mauch PM, Kalish LA, Kadin M, et al. Patterns of presentation of Hodgkin disease. Implications for etiology and pathogenesis. *Cancer* 1993; 71:2062.

[35] Kaplan HS. Hodgkin's Disease, 2nd ed, Harvard University Press, Cambridge, MA 1980.

[36] Gobbi PG, Cavalli C, Gendarini A, et al. Reevaluation of prognostic significance of symptoms in Hodgkin's disease. *Cancer* 1985; 56:2874.

[37] Atkinson K, Austin DE, McElwain TJ, Peckham MJ. Alcohol pain in Hodgkin's disease. *Cancer* 1976; 37:895.

[38] Lucker GP, Steijlen PM. Acrokeratosisparaneoplastica (Bazex syndrome) occurring with acquired ichthyosis in Hodgkin's disease. *Br. J. Dermatol.* 1995; 133:322.

[39] Perifanis V, Sfikas G, Tziomalos K, et al. Skin involvement in Hodgkin's disease. *Cancer Invest.* 2006; 24:401.

[40] Seymour JF, Gagel RF. Calcitriol: the major humoral mediator of hypercalcemia in Hodgkin's disease and non-Hodgkin's lymphomas. *Blood* 1993; 82:1383.

[41] Rieke JW, Donaldson SS, Horning SJ. Hypercalcemia and vitamin D metabolism in Hodgkin's disease. Is there an underlying immunoregulatory relationship? *Cancer* 1989; 63:1700.

[42] Shah SJ, Warrier RP, Ode DL, et al. Immune thrombocytopenia and hemolytic anemia associated with Hodgkin disease. *J. Pediatr. Hematol. Oncol.* 1996; 18:227.

[43] Sierra RD. Coombs-positive hemolytic anemia in Hodgkin's disease: case presentation and review of the literature. *Mil. Med.* 1991; 156:691.

[44] Di Biagio E, Sánchez-Borges M, Desenne JJ, et al. Eosinophilia in Hodgkin's disease: a role for interleukin 5. *Int. Arch. Allergy Immunol.* 1996; 110:244.

[45] Teruya-Feldstein J, Jaffe ES, Burd PR, et al. Differential chemokine expression in tissues involved by Hodgkin's disease: direct correlation of eotaxin expression and tissue eosinophilia. *Blood* 1999; 93:2463.

[46] Peters MV, Alison RE, Bush RS. Natural history of Hodgkin's disease as related to staging. *Cancer* 1966; 19; 308.

[47] Castellino, R.A., Hodgkin disease: practical concepts for the diagnostic radiologist. *Radiology*, 1986. 159(2): p. 305-10.

[48] Castellino, R.A., et al., Hodgkin disease: contributions of chest CT in the initial staging evaluation. *Radiology*, 1986. 160(3): p. 603-5.

[49] Castellani, M.R., et al., Gallium scan in adolescents and children with Hodgkin's disease (HL). Treatment response assessment and prognostic value. *Q. J. Nucl. Med.*, 2003. 47(1): p. 22-30.

[50] Friedberg, J.W., et al., FDG-PET is superior to gallium scintigraphy in staging and more sensitive in the follow-up of patients with de novo Hodgkin lymphoma: a blinded comparison. *Leuk. Lymphoma*, 2004. 45(1): p. 85-92.

[51] Hudson, M.M., M.J. Krasin, and S.C. Kaste, PET imaging in pediatric Hodgkin's lymphoma. *Pediatr. Radiol.*, 2004. 34(3): p. 190-8.

[52] Kaste, S.C., et al., 18F-FDG-avid sites mimicking active disease in pediatric Hodgkin's. *Pediatr. Radiol.*, 2005. 35(2): p. 141-54.

[53] Lister, T.A. and D. Crowther, Staging for Hodgkin's disease. *Semin. Oncol.*, 1990. 17(6): p. 696-703.

[54] Carbone, P.P., et al., Report of the Committee on Hodgkin's Disease Staging Classification. *Cancer Res.*, 1971. 31(11): p. 1860-1.

[55] Lister TA, Crowther D, Sutcliffe SB, et al. Report of a committee convened to discuss the evaluation and staging of patients with Hodgkin's disease: Cotswolds meeting. *J. Clin. Oncol.* 1989; 7:1630.
[56] Jost LM, Stahel RA; ESMO Guidelines Task Force.: ESMO Minimum Clinical Recommendations for diagnosis, treatment and follow-up of Hodgkin's disease. *Ann. Oncol.* 16 (Suppl 1): i54-5, 2005.
[57] Hasenclever D, Diehl V: A prognostic score for advanced Hodgkin's disease. International Prognostic Factors Project on Advanced Hodgkin's Disease. *N. Engl. J. Med.* 339 (21): 1506-14, 1998.
[58] Shankar, A.G., et al., Does histology influence outcome in childhood Hodgkin's disease? Results from the United Kingdom Children's Cancer Study Group. *J. Clin. Oncol.*, 1997. 15(7): p. 2622-30.
[59] Christiansen, I., et al., Soluble vascular cell adhesion molecule-1 (sVCAM-1) is an independent prognostic marker in Hodgkin's disease. *Br. J. Haematol.*, 1998. 102(3): p. 701-9.
[60] Chronowski, G.M., et al., An elevated serum beta-2-microglobulin level is an adverse prognostic factor for overall survival in patients with early-stage Hodgkin disease. *Cancer*, 2002. 95(12): p. 2534-8.
[61] Nadali, G., et al., Serum level of the soluble form of the CD30 molecule identifies patients with Hodgkin's disease at high risk of unfavorable outcome. *Blood*, 1998. 91(8): p. 3011-6.
[62] Warzocha, K., et al., Plasma levels of tumour necrosis factor and its soluble receptors correlate with clinical features and outcome of Hodgkin's disease patients. *Br. J. Cancer*, 1998. 77(12): p. 2357-62.
[63] Dukers, D.F., et al., High numbers of active caspase 3-positive Reed-Sternberg cells in pretreatment biopsy specimens of patients with Hodgkin disease predict favorable clinical outcome. *Blood*, 2002. 100(1): p. 36-42.
[64] Carde, P., et al., Early response to chemotherapy: a surrogate for final outcome of Hodgkin's disease patients that should influence initial treatment length and intensity? *Ann. Oncol.*, 2002. 13 Suppl 1: p. 86-91.
[65] Landman-Parker, J., et al., Localized childhood Hodgkin's disease: response-adapted chemotherapy with etoposide, bleomycin, vinblastine, and prednisone before low-dose radiation therapy-results of the French Society of Pediatric Oncology Study MDH90. *J. Clin. Oncol.*, 2000. 18(7): p. 1500-7.
[66] Schwartz C, C.L., London W, Intensive response based therapy with or without dexrazoxane for intermediate/high stage (I/HS) pediatric Hodgkin's disease (HL): a Pediatric Oncology Group (POG) Study, in Fifth International Symposium on Hodgkin's lymphoma, A.J. Polliack A, Diehl V et al, Editor. 2001, Harwood Academic: Koln, Germany.
[67] Smith RA, C.Q., Hudson M, et al, Prognostic factors in pediatric Hodgkin's disease. *J. Radiat. Oncol. Biol. Phys.*, 2001. 51(3 Suppl 1): p. 119.
[68] Nachman, J.B., et al., Randomized comparison of low-dose involved-field radiotherapy and no radiotherapy for children with Hodgkin's disease who achieve a complete response to chemotherapy. *J. Clin. Oncol.*, 2002. 20(18): p. 3765-71.
[69] Gallamini, A., et al., Early interim 2-[18F]fluoro-2-deoxy-D-glucose positron emission tomography is prognostically superior to international prognostic score in advanced-

stage Hodgkin's lymphoma: a report from a joint Italian-Danish study. *J. Clin. Oncol.*, 2007. 25(24): p. 3746-52.

[70] Hutchings, M., et al., FDG-PET after two cycles of chemotherapy predicts treatment failure and progression-free survival in Hodgkin lymphoma. *Blood*, 2006. 107(1): p. 52-9.

[71] Sears JD, Greven KM, Ferree CR, et al.: Definitive irradiation in the treatment of Hodgkin's disease. Analysis of outcome, prognostic factors, and long-term complications. *Cancer* 79 (1): 145-51, 1997.

[72] Ng AK, Mauch PM: Radiation therapy in Hodgkin's lymphoma. SeminHematol 36 (3): 290-302, 1999.

[73] Dühmke E, Franklin J, Pfreundschuh M, et al.: Low-dose radiation is sufficient for the noninvolved extended-field treatment in favorable early-stage Hodgkin's disease: long-term results of a randomized trial of radiotherapy alone. *J. Clin. Oncol.* 19 (11): 2905-14, 2001.

[74] Mendenhall NP, Rodrigue LL, Moore-Higgs GJ, et al.: The optimal dose of radiation in Hodgkin's disease: an analysis of clinical and treatment factors affecting in-field disease control. *Int. J. Radiat. Oncol. Biol. Phys.* 44 (3): 551-61, 1999.

[75] Fermé C, Eghbali H, Meerwaldt JH, et al.: Chemotherapy plus involved-field radiation in early-stage Hodgkin's disease. *N. Engl. J. Med.* 357 (19): 1916-27, 2007.

[76] Meyer RM, Gospodarowicz MK, Connors JM, et al.: Randomized comparison of ABVD chemotherapy with a strategy that includes radiation therapy in patients with limited-stage Hodgkin's lymphoma: National Cancer Institute of Canada Clinical Trials Group and the Eastern Cooperative Oncology Group. *J. Clin. Oncol.* 23 (21): 4634-42, 2005.

[77] Tubiana M, Henry-Amar M, Carde P, et al.: Toward comprehensive management tailored to prognostic factors of patients with clinical stages I and II in Hodgkin's disease. The EORTC Lymphoma Group controlled clinical trials: 1964-1987. *Blood* 73 (1): 47-56, 1989.

[78] Diehl V, Brillant C, Engert A, et al.: Recent interim analysis of the HD11 trial of the GHSG: intensification of chemotherapy and reduction of radiation dose in early unfavorable stage Hodgkin's lymphoma. [Abstract] *Blood* 106 (11): A-816, 2005.

[79] Eich HT, Diehl V, Görgen H, et al.: Intensified chemotherapy and dose-reduced involved-field radiotherapy in patients with early unfavorable Hodgkin's lymphoma: final analysis of the German Hodgkin Study Group HD11 trial. *J. Clin. Oncol.* 28 (27): 4199-206, 2010.

[80] Noordijk EM, Thomas J, Fermé C, et al.: First results of the EORTC-GELA H9 randomized trials: the H9-F trial (comparing 3 radiation dose levels) and H9-U trial (comparing 3 chemotherapy schemes) in patients with favorable or unfavorable early stage Hodgkin's lymphoma (HL) . [Abstract] *J. Clin. Oncol.* 23 (Suppl 16): A-6505, 561s, 2005.

[81] Hasenclever D, Diehl V: A prognostic score for advanced Hodgkin's disease. International Prognostic Factors Project on Advanced Hodgkin's Disease. *N. Engl. J. Med.* 339 (21): 1506-14, 1998.

[82] Canellos GP, Anderson JR, Propert KJ, et al.: Chemotherapy of advanced Hodgkin's disease with MOPP, ABVD, or MOPP alternating with ABVD. *N. Engl. J. Med.* 327 (21): 1478-84, 1992.

[83] Federico M, Luminari S, Iannitto E, et al.: ABVD compared with BEACOPP compared with CEC for the initial treatment of patients with advanced Hodgkin's lymphoma: results from the HD2000 Gruppo Italiano per lo Studio dei Linfomi Trial. *J. Clin. Oncol.* 27 (5): 805-11, 2009.

[84] Engert A, Diehl V, Franklin J, et al.: Escalated-dose BEACOPP in the treatment of patients with advanced-stage Hodgkin's lymphoma: 10 years of follow-up of the GHSG HD9 study. *J. Clin. Oncol.* 27 (27): 4548-54, 2009.

[85] Federico M, Bellei M, Brice P, et al.: High-dose therapy and autologous stem-cell transplantation versus conventional therapy for patients with advanced Hodgkin's lymphoma responding to front-line therapy. *J. Clin. Oncol*. 21 (12): 2320-5, 2003.

[86] Bhatia, S., et al., Breast cancer and other second neoplasms after childhood Hodgkin's disease. *N. Engl. J. Med.*, 1996. 334(12): p. 745-51.

[87] Hancock, S.L., S.S. Donaldson, and R.T. Hoppe, Cardiac disease following treatment of Hodgkin's disease in children and adolescents. *J. Clin. Oncol.*, 1993. 11(7): p. 1208-15.

[88] Donaldson, S.S. and M.P. Link, Combined modality treatment with low-dose radiation and MOPP chemotherapy for children with Hodgkin's disease. *J. Clin. Oncol.*, 1987. 5(5): p. 742-9.

[89] Hutchinson, R.J., et al., MOPP or radiation in addition to ABVD in the treatment of pathologically staged advanced Hodgkin's disease in children: results of the Children's Cancer Group Phase III Trial. *J. Clin. Oncol.*, 1998. 16(3): p. 897-906.

[90] Weiner, M.A., et al., Randomized study of intensive MOPP-ABVD with or without low-dose total-nodal radiation therapy in the treatment of stages IIB, IIIA2, IIIB, and IV Hodgkin's disease in pediatric patients: a Pediatric Oncology Group study. *J. Clin. Oncol.*, 1997. 15(8): p. 2769-79.

[91] Beaty, O., 3rd, et al., Subsequent malignancies in children and adolescents after treatment for Hodgkin's disease. *J. Clin. Oncol.*, 1995. 13(3): p. 603-9.

[92] Nogová L, Reineke T, Brillant C, et al. Lymphocyte-predominant and classical Hodgkin's lymphoma: a comprehensive analysis from the German Hodgkin Study Group. *J. Clin. Oncol.* 2008; 26:434.

[93] Miettinen M, Franssila KO, Saxén E. Hodgkin's disease, lymphocytic predominance nodular. Increased risk for subsequent non-Hodgkin's lymphomas. *Cancer* 1983; 51:2293.

[94] Hansmann ML, Zwingers T, Böske A, et al. Clinical features of nodular paragranuloma (Hodgkin's disease, lymphocyte predominance type, nodular). *J. Cancer Res. Clin. Oncol.* 1984; 108:321.

[95] Pellegrino B, Terrier-Lacombe MJ, Oberlin O, et al. Lymphocyte-predominant Hodgkin's lymphoma in children: therapeutic abstention after initial lymph node resection--a Study of the French Society of Pediatric Oncology. *J. Clin. Oncol.* 2003; 21:2948.

[96] Murphy SB, Morgan ER, Katzenstein HM, Kletzel M. Results of little or no treatment for lymphocyte-predominant Hodgkin disease in children and adolescents. *J. Pediatr. Hematol. Oncol.* 2003; 25:684.

[97] Mauz-Körholz C, Gorde-Grosjean S, Hasenclever D, et al. Resection alone in 58 children with limited stage, lymphocyte-predominant Hodgkin lymphoma-experience from the European network group on pediatric Hodgkin lymphoma. *Cancer* 2007; 110:179.

[98] Wirth A, Yuen K, Barton M, et al. Long-term outcome after radiotherapy alone for lymphocyte-predominant Hodgkin lymphoma: a retrospective multicenter study of the Australasian Radiation Oncology Lymphoma Group. *Cancer* 2005; 104:1221.
[99] Cannellos G.P., What is appopriate systemic chemotherapy for lymphocyte predominant Hodgkin lymphoma?. *J. Clin. Oncol.*, 2009. 28(1): p. e8.
[100] Lieskovsky, Y.E., et al., High-dose therapy and autologous hematopoietic stem-cell transplantation for recurrent or refractory pediatric Hodgkin's disease: results and prognostic indices. *J. Clin. Oncol.*, 2004. 22(22): p. 4532-40.
[101] Bhatia, S., et al., High risk of subsequent neoplasms continues with extended follow-up of childhood Hodgkin's disease: report from the Late Effects Study Group. *J. Clin. Oncol.*, 2003. 21(23): p. 4386-94.
[102] Green, D.M., et al., Second malignant neoplasms after treatment for Hodgkin's disease in childhood or adolescence. *J. Clin. Oncol.*, 2000. 18(7): p. 1492-9.
[103] Metayer, C., et al., Second cancers among long-term survivors of Hodgkin's disease diagnosed in childhood and adolescence. *J. Clin. Oncol.*, 2000. 18(12): p. 2435-43.
[104] van Leeuwen, F.E., et al., Long-term risk of second malignancy in survivors of Hodgkin's disease treated during adolescence or young adulthood. *J. Clin. Oncol.*, 2000. 18(3): p. 487-97.
[105] Wolden, S.L., et al., Second cancers following pediatric Hodgkin's disease. *J. Clin. Oncol.*, 1998. 16(2): p. 536-44.
[106] Josting, A., et al., Secondary myeloid leukemia and myelodysplastic syndromes in patients treated for Hodgkin's disease: a report from the German Hodgkin's Lymphoma Study Group. *J. Clin. Oncol.*, 2003. 21(18): p. 3440-6.
[107] Neglia, J.P., et al., Second malignant neoplasms in five-year survivors of childhood cancer: childhood cancer survivor study. *J. Natl. Cancer Inst.*, 2001. 93(8): p. 618-29.
[108] Kenney, L.B., et al., Breast cancer after childhood cancer: a report from the Childhood Cancer Survivor Study. *Ann. Intern. Med.*, 2004. 141(8): p. 590-7.
[109] Travis, L.B., et al., Breast cancer following radiotherapy and chemotherapy among young women with Hodgkin disease. *JAMA*, 2003. 290(4): p. 465-75.
[110] Adams, M.J., et al., Cardiovascular status in long-term survivors of Hodgkin's disease treated with chest radiotherapy. *J. Clin. Oncol.*, 2004. 22(15): p. 3139-48.
[111] Ewer, M.S., et al., Doxorubicin cardiotoxicity in children: comparison of a consecutive divided daily dose administration schedule with single dose (rapid) infusion administration. *Med. Pediatr. Oncol.*, 1998. 31(6): p. 512-5.
[112] Grenier, M.A. and S.E. Lipshultz, Epidemiology of anthracycline cardiotoxicity in children and adults. *Semin. Oncol.*, 1998. 25(4 Suppl 10): p. 72-85.
[113] Krischer, J.P., et al., Clinical cardiotoxicity following anthracycline treatment for childhood cancer: the Pediatric Oncology Group experience. *J. Clin. Oncol.*, 1997. 15(4): p. 1544-52.
[114] Lipshultz, S.E., et al., Doxorubicin administration by continuous infusion is not cardioprotective: the Dana-Farber 91-01 Acute Lymphoblastic Leukemia protocol. *J. Clin. Oncol.*, 2002. 20(6): p. 1677-82.
[115] Lipshultz, S.E., et al., Long-term enalapril therapy for left ventricular dysfunction in doxorubicin-treated survivors of childhood cancer. *J. Clin. Oncol.*, 2002. 20(23): p. 4517-22.

[116] Lipshultz, S.E., et al., Monitoring for anthracycline cardiotoxicity. *Pediatrics*, 1994. 93(3): p. 433-7.

[117] Nysom, K., et al., Relationship between cumulative anthracycline dose and late cardiotoxicity in childhood acute lymphoblastic leukemia. *J. Clin. Oncol.*, 1998. 16(2): p. 545-50.

[118] Pein, F., et al., Cardiac abnormalities 15 years and more after adriamycin therapy in 229 childhood survivors of a solid tumour at the Institut Gustave Roussy. *Br. J. Cancer*, 2004. 91(1): p. 37-44.

[119] Silber, J.H., et al., Increased risk of cardiac dysfunction after anthracyclines in girls. *Med. Pediatr. Oncol.*, 1993. 21(7): p. 477-9.

[120] Steinherz, L.J., et al., Guidelines for cardiac monitoring of children during and after anthracycline therapy: report of the Cardiology Committee of the Childrens Cancer Study Group. *Pediatrics*, 1992. 89(5 Pt 1): p. 942-9.

[121] Bossi, G., et al., Long-term pulmonary sequelae after treatment of childhood Hodgkin's disease. *Ann. Oncol.*, 1997. 8 Suppl 1: p. 19-24.

[122] Fryer, C.J., et al., Efficacy and toxicity of 12 courses of ABVD chemotherapy followed by low-dose regional radiation in advanced Hodgkin's disease in children: a report from the Children's Cancer Study Group. *J. Clin. Oncol.*, 1990. 8(12): p. 1971-80.

[123] Kreisman, H. and N. Wolkove, Pulmonary toxicity of antineoplastic therapy. *Semin. Oncol.*, 1992. 19(5): p. 508-20.

[124] Gleeson, H.K., K. Darzy, and S.M. Shalet, Late endocrine, metabolic and skeletal sequelae following treatment of childhood cancer. *Best Pract. Res. Clin. Endocrinol. Metab.*, 2002. 16(2): p. 335-48.

[125] Sklar, C., et al., Abnormalities of the thyroid in survivors of Hodgkin's disease: data from the Childhood Cancer Survivor Study. *J. Clin. Endocrinol. Metab.*, 2000. 85(9): p. 3227-32.

[126] Hill, M., et al., Evaluation of the efficacy of the VEEP regimen in adult Hodgkin's disease with assessment of gonadal and cardiac toxicity. *J. Clin. Oncol.*, 1995. 13(2): p. 387-95.

[127] Relander, T., et al., Gonadal and sexual function in men treated for childhood cancer. *Med. Pediatr. Oncol.*, 2000. 35(1): p. 52-63.

[128] Ash, P., The influence of radiation on fertility in man. *Br. J. Radiol.*, 1980. 53(628): p. 271-8.

[129] Byrne, J., Infertility and premature menopause in childhood cancer survivors. *Med. Pediatr. Oncol.*, 1999. 33(1): p. 24-8.

[130] Haukvik, U.K., et al., Treatment-related premature ovarian failure as a long-term complication after Hodgkin's lymphoma. *Ann. Oncol.*, 2006. 17(9): p. 1428-33.

ND

In: Hodgkin's and T-Cell Lymphoma
Editors: Warren K. Harvey and Randall M. Jacobs
ISBN 978-1-62257-478-0

Chapter 4

HODGKIN'S LYMPHOMA: PATHOGENESIS, DIAGNOSIS, TREATMENT OPTIONS AND PROGNOSIS

***Árpád Illés*[1,*], *Ádám Jóna*[1], *László Váróczy*[1], *Zsófia Miltényi*[1], *Zsófia Simon*[1] *and Peter Szodoray*[2]**
[1]3rd Department of Medicine, Institute for Medicine;
University of Debrecen Medical and Health Science Center,
Debrecen, Hungary;
[2]Institute of Immunology, Rikshospitalet,
Oslo University Hospital, Oslo, Norway

ABSTRACT

Hodgkin's lymphoma (HL) is a rare monoclonal lymphoid malignancy of B-cell origin, which represents circa 12-18 % of all lymphomas.

It shows characteristic clinical and morphological features. The disease remains localised for a long period of time. The histological characteristics are the bilobated Hodgkin and Reed-Sternberg (HRS) cells for classical HL, and their variants the lymphocytic and hystiocytic (LandH) cells, for nodular lymphocyte predominant HL, surrounded by large, non-malignant, reactive tissue. Both pathognomonic HRS and LandH cells go through somatic hypermutation. Phenotypically HRS cells are CD15 and CD30 positive, while LandH cells are CD20 positive. The exact etiology is still unknown, however the role of genetical, immunological and viral infection (Ebstein-Barr virus) seem important. Environmental factors might explain, why deficient response against HRS cells occurs. More than half of the HL patients have no complaints, lymphadenomegaly and hepato-splenomegaly can be seen at the time of the diagnosis, while B symptoms (fever, night sweats and loss of weight) are more specific for advanced stage. Patients suspect to HL go through a specific check-up, lymph node and bone marrow biopsy for histological diagnosis and various imaging techniques (ultrasound, X-ray, CT or, ^{18}FDG PET/CT scan) for staging. Nowadays the standard

* ÁRPÁD ILLÉS MD, PhD. 3rd Department of Medicine, University of Debrecen, Móricz Zs. 22., H-4022 Debrecen, Hungary, Phone: +36 52 255 218, Fax: +36 52 255 218. Email: illesarpaddr@gmail.com

combined chemo-radiotherapy consisting of adriamycin bleomycin vinblastine dacarbazine (ABVD) regimen is expected to cure 80-85% of patients. Risk-adapted strategy involving conventional prognostic factors, such as the European Organization for Research and Treatment of Cancer (EORTC), in early and International Prognostic Score (IPS) in advanced stage HL are known to avoid over- and under-treating patients. The early identification of refractory patients by interim PET/CT may be beneficial thus further improves patient outcome and help to avoid late side effects. Combining standard care with novel epigenetic and targeted therapies (anti-CD20 and anti-CD30 antibodies) may be promising and clinical trials currently take place to assess the efficacy of these novel treatment regimes.

General Features

Hodgkin's lymphoma (HL) represents 12-18% of all lymphomas, it shows characteristic clinical, morphological and therapeutic features. The pathognomonic Hodgkin cells and its variants the bilobated Reed-Sternberg cells in classical HL and lymphocytic and hystiocytic (LandH) cells in nodular lymphocyte predominant HL are proven to be of B-cell origin. Several factors are known to play a role in the development of HL, including Epstein-Barr viral infection, genetic and immunological factors, however unknown agents may also play a role in the pathomechanism. HL is one of the best treatable oncological diseases: current standard of care is expected to cure 80-85% of patients.

Histological Classification

The latest World Health Organization (WHO) classification distinguishes two subgroups of HL, the nodular lymphocyte predominant HL (NLPHL) and classical HL (cHL), based on pathogenesis, morphological appearance, immunophenotype and clinical characteristics.

The affected lymph nodes show at least partially nodular characteristics in NLPHL, tumor cells are known to be lymphocytic and hystiocytic (LandH) cells, as well as so-called popcorn cells. In contrast, tumor cells are Hodgkin, Reed-Sternberg (HRS) and lacunar cells in cHL, which can be further subdivided into four subgroups: lymphocyte rich (cLR), mixed cellularity (cMC), nodular sclerosis (cNS) and lymphocyte depletion subgroups (cLD). In some cases a subgroup cannot be determined (ND), in other cases histology (and clinical features) shows intermediate disease between cNS and primary mediastinal large B cell lymphoma (PMBCL), which is known as a novel entity in the current WHO classification [1].

Etiology

Although the B cell origin of HRS cells is well known, the pathomechanism is not yet clearly defined. Endogenous and environmental factors may collectively contribute to the development of HL [2].

Risk and provoking factors are:

- Endogenous factors are suspected since the occurrence of HL is hundred fold in homozygous twins compared to heterozygous twins. A clear genetic variation, which contributes to the pathogenesis of HL, cannot be detected [3].
- Immunological factors are suspected since cellular immunodeficiency and immunoregulatory disorders are detectable both in untreated, cured patients, as well as patients in remission. Moreover, HL is more frequent in immunodeficient conditions, including AIDS and transplanted patients with continuous immunosuppression. The risk of HL is fifty fold in autoimmune-lymphoproliferative syndrome, characterized by CD95/Fas mutation [4].
- Several epidemiological data imply, that an infective agent may contribute to the development of HL. The etiological role of Epstein-Barr virus (EBV) is verified in the following cases:
    - cHL is 3 times more frequent in those, who underwent infectious mononucleosis in adulthood
    - Anti-EBV titer is higher in HL patients
    - Clonal EBV genome and its product, latent membrane protein (LMP1, 2) can be detected in 20-80% of cHL patients in the pathognomonic HRS cells (especially in the cMC subgroup in childhood and late adulthood), though NLPHL cases are negative. The clonality of the EBV genome refers to, that HL develops from one single cell [2].

LMP1 increases Bcl2 expression, the generation of certain cytokines and activates NF-κB. LMP2a helps avoiding B cells from apoptosis even if they do not express a B cell receptor (Ig gene is not functional). These events might explain the development of cHL in certain EBV positive cases, however the "hit and run mechanism" of EBV and the etiological role of other lymphotrop viruses could not be confirmed in EBV negative cases [5].

Pathogenesis

Reactive microenvironment may play a key role in the survival of HRS cells [6]. HRS cells express a variety of antigens on their surface (CD15, Pax5, CD20, MUM1, CD138, CD30, etc.) which helps them maintaining molecular mimicry and anti-apoptotic phenotype [7]. Gene expression profiling revealed down-regulation of the genes of B cell phenotype, which includes numerous cell surface molecules (CD22, CD52), members of the signalling pathways (Syk, Blk) and transcription factors (Oct-2, Bob1, Pu.1) [6, 8]. This also leads to the lack of Ig expression. Other factors are also responsible for abnormal differentiation (E2A, Pax5, Notch1) [9-11].Janus kinase-signal transducer and activator of transcription (JAK-STAT), nuclear factor-κB (NF-κB) and phophatidilinositol 3-kinase-Akt (PI3K-Akt) pathways are often reported to be involved in the survival of HRS cells. *(Figure 1)* Somatic mutation of NF-κB inhibitor IκBalpha and genomic amplification of c-Rel gene lead to the constitutive activations of NF-κB [6, 12]. cFLIP and XIAP, the target genes of NF-κB might be responsible for inhibiting CD95 and TRAIL mediated apoptosis. [13, 14] LMP1, which can be detectable in EBV infected HRS cells also activate NF-κB. LMP2a, another viral molecule, imitates B cell receptor, might play a role in avoiding apoptosis, as well.

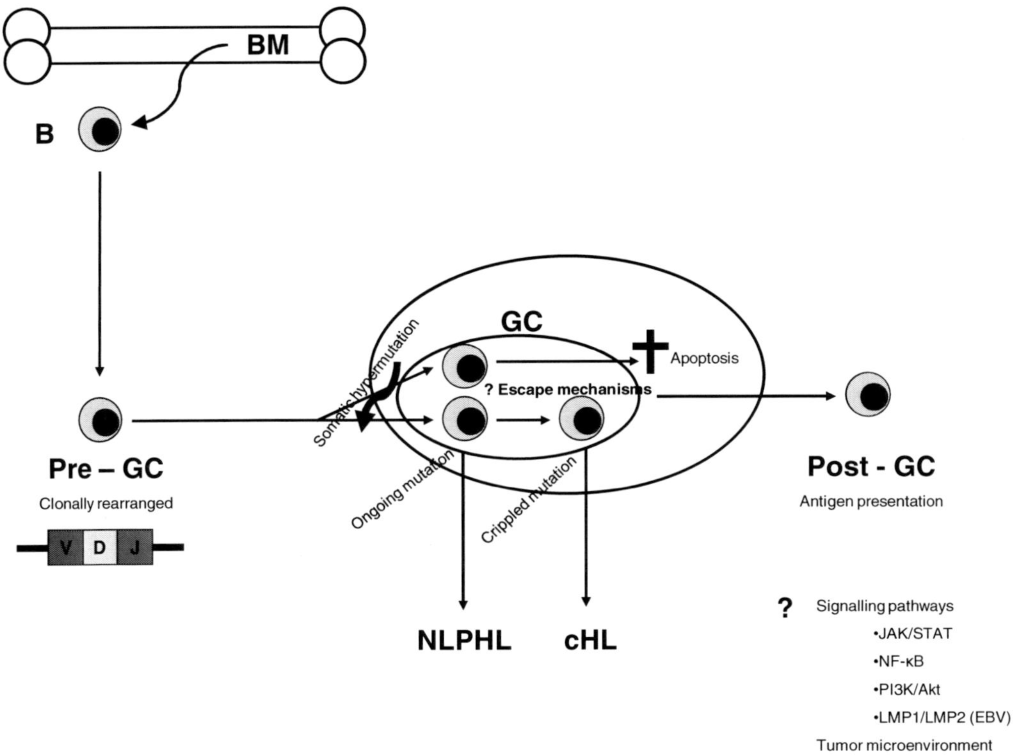

Figure 1. The possible pathomechanism of Hodgkin's lymphoma.

BM – bone marrow, GC – germinal center, NLPHL - nodular lymphocyte predominant Hodgkin's lymphoma, HL – Hodgkin's lymphoma.

Once HRS cells are present, it is crucial that they have to be surrounded by an appropriate microenvironment, which includes lymphocytes, macrophages, eosinophils, plasma cells and fibroblasts. It has been reported previously, that such microenvironment is essential to avoid any effective immune response against HRS cells. This includes a shift from T-helper 1 towards T-helper 2 immune response [15]. Particular changes in secretion of citokines/chemokines have been described, including Regulated on Activation Normal T cell Expressed and Secreted (RANTES), Thymus and Activation Regulated Chemokine (TARC), interleukin (IL)-5, IL-6, IL-9, IL-10 and IL-13. HRS cells also express immunosuppressive factors such as IL-10, transforming growth factor (TGF)-β, galectin-1 and prostaglandin E2 [16].The molecular, cellular background, as well as the role of the tumor microenvironment is of special interest as part of the development of new biological prognostic factors and targets for novel therapies [17].

Genetic Background

A typical genetic abnormality contributing to the pathogenesis of HL cannot be detected, contrary to several non-Hodgkin's lymphoma (NHL) subtypes, although aberration of several chromosomes and chromosome regions were observed in certain HRS cells.

Loss on one allele in the 4q26 region and defect of a tumor suppressor gene in the 6q25 region may play an important role in the development of cHL [18]. Comparative gene hybridization revealed aberrations at the 2p, 9q and 12q regions, while fluorescent in situ hybridization (FISH) revealed amplifications of JAK42 genes at the 9p23-24 loci and of the MDM2 gene at the 12q14 loci, which play an important role in apoptosis inhibition [19, 20]. Another genomic instability was discovered at the 2p13-16 region, which may lead to the constitutive activation of NF-κB and STAT, leading to resistance to apoptosis [21, 22]. Most recently the aberration of the 16p11-13 loci has been shown to correlate with resistance to therapy [23].

Gene expression profiling of HRS cell cultures revealed that they are most similar to activated B cells. Twenty-seven genes were over-expressed, while 45 genes were downregulated, including both pro-apoptotic (CD95) and anti-apoptotic (NF-κB, TRAF1, cIAP1, cFLIP) molecules. Remarkable aberrations of various transcription factors are identified, which can be excellent novel therapeutic targets, yet their exact role in the pathogenesis is still unknown [24]. The origin of immunoregulatory disorders is unclear. Interestingly, the risk of HL is fifty fold in autoimmune-lymphoproliferative syndrome, related to CD95/Fas mutation [4]. Although familiar cases have been described, they are extremely rare.

EPIDEMIOLOGY

HL occurs worldwide, its international incidence (except for Asia, where its relatively rare [25]) shows low bias in both genders. In the United States HL represents about 11.4% of all lymphomas [26], while the incidence rate is 2.2/100 000. There is an estimated 9060 new HL cases prognosed in 2012; 4960 for males and 4100 for females. [27] NLPHL represents about 3-6% of all HL cases [28]. A slight (1.2-1.5:1) male predominance can be seen, with a bimodal age-pattern and incidence peak between 20-30 and 50-60 years of age. There are certain variances in geographical and socio-economic features of HL patients. At the first incidence peak moderate female and significant cNS predominance can be observed. In developing countries the incidence peak is in childhood with characteristic advanced stage and cMC subtype, while in early adulthood, cNS subtype and early stage is characteristic for the developed countries [29].

CLINICAL PATHOLOGICAL FEATURES

Classical Hodgkin's Lymphoma

In classical HL, the ratio of tumor cells (HRS, lacunar, LandH cells) is low, which are surrounded by a non-malignant, reactive cell mass, consisting of epitheloid cells, histyocytes, lymphocytes, eosinophyl granulocytes, and plasma cells. Tumor cells are frequently surrounded by T cells in a rosette shape [30].

At the time of the diagnosis, patients have no specific complaints; enlarged lymph nodes in the neck, or mediastinum are characteristic. Less frequently, any lymph node region might be enlarged. Systemic (B-symptoms) are specific for the advanced stage (fever, loss weight, night sweats). Fever is usually undulant (Pel-Ebstein fever), and itching is troublesome.

The disease continuously spreads through the lymph node regions. The disease appears more frequently above the diaphragm; the cervical, or supraclavicular regions are affected in 60-80% of cases, while the mediastinal region is affected in about half of the cases.

The mediastinal region is often "bulky size", which spreads directly to the lungs, pericardia, and the chest. Under the diaphragm, the celiac lymph node regions are affected at first, later it progresses typically to the para-aortic and pelvic regions.

Extranodal manifestations are less frequent, compared to non-Hodgkin's lymphomas, and the spleen is the most frequent location. Usually it spreads from nodal to extranodal regions, however hematogenous spreading might also occur. Bone marrow is infiltrated in 8-15% of the cases, which is more frequent in the advanced stage with B-symptoms, resulting in pancytopenia. The disease usually affects the younger population, it has common co morbidities: immunodeficient conditions (mostly cellular), which contribute to frequent bacterial and unusual fungal and viral infections. Immunothrobocytopenia (ITP), autoimmune hemolytic anemia (AIHA), nephrosis, skin symptoms (vasculitis, pemphigus), neurological disorders (e.g. limbic encephalopathy, subacute cerebellar degeneration) may be also present [31-33].

Nodular Lymphocyte Predominant Hodgkin's Lymphoma

Most frequently it develops in young males, usually has a peripheral (cervical) location.

Bulky tumor is not characteristic to NLPHL, while the clinical picture is similar to indolent lymphomas. CD20 positive tumor cells are present. Patients relapse more often, however the overall survival is better. NLPHL might transform to diffuse large B cell lymphoma (DLBCL).

Table 1. Features of classical (cHL) and nodular lymphocyte predominant Hodgkin lymphoma (NLPHL)

	cHL	NLPHL
Age pattern	Bimodal	Unimodal
Male ratio	NS: 50%, MC 70%	70%
Localization	Mediastinum, abdomen, spleen	Peripheral lymph nodes
Stage at time of diagnosis	II. or III-IV.	I. or II.
B-symptoms	40 %	<20 %
Clinical behavior	Aggressive	Indolent, late relapses
Risk of DLCBL	1%	2-6.5%

Staging

Clinical staging is performed according to the Ann Arbor Classification and Cotswold's modification [33-35].

Stage I.: A single lymph node region or organ is affected
Stage II.: Two or more lymph node region or organ are affected localized on the same side of the diaphragm
Stage III.: Affected lymph nodes on both sides of the diaphragm
III/1.: portal, hilar-spleen and celiac
III/2.: paraaortic, mesenteric, iliacal, inguinal lymph node regions are affected
Stage IV.: disseminated, diffuse extranodal involvement, indirect development

Further classification can be made based on the lack (A) or the presence (B) of general symptoms: fever (>38 °C), weight loss (more than 10% of weight in the past 6 months), night sweats. "X" means bulky disease, which is considered more than one third of the diameter of the diaphragm or more than 10 cm or diameter of lymph node conglomerate more than 5 cm anywhere in the body. "E" means unifocal direct involvement of an organ (contradictory to St. IV, indirect extranodal involvement).

Diagnosis

Histological and immunohistological assessment is needed for the correct diagnosis, while cytology alone is insufficient. The WHO classification distinguishes cHL and NLPHL based on the pathogenesis, morphological appearance, immunophenotype and clinical characteristics. In NLPHL the affected lymph nodes have at least partially nodular characteristics. Tumor cells are LandH cells and popcorn cells, which are CD19, CD20, CD22, CD79a, Bcl-6, J-chain, CD45 and EMA positive. In contrast tumor cells in cHL (HRS, lacunar cells) are CD15 and CD30 positive but negative for B-cell markers [30].

Necessary investigations

- Past medical history
- Physical examination (affected lymph node regions, liver and spleen size in cm)
- Ear-nose-throat (ENT) examination
- Lab tests (blood count, erythrocyte sedimentation rate, kidney, liver function, lactate dehydrogenase (LDH), alcalic phophatase, viral tests (HIV, hepatitis), Coombs test
- Bone marrow biopsy is obligatory is advanced stages and with blood count disorders (Evidence I/A)
- Chest X-ray, abdominal and pelvic ultrasound, computed tomography (CT) scan (cervical, thoracal, abdominal, pelvic) (Evidence I/A) or 18 Fluoro-deoxy-glucose positron emission tomography (18FDG PET) CT which is considered to be the current standard (Evidence I/A-B) [36] (7)
- Staging laparatomy is not recommended (Evidence II/A)

Other possible examinations

- Magnetic resonance imaging (MRI) - nervous system and epidural localization, bone disorders
- Endoscopy
- Electrocardiography, echocardiography (patients with anthracyclin therapy),
- Lung functional test
- Andrological examination for males, sperm cryopreservation [31, 33].
- For females *in vitro* fertilization followed by embryo cryopreservation is widely available, however it may postpone therapy. Oocyte cryopreservation is still an experimental technique [37].

Differential diagnosis

HL should be differentiated from several conditions, which appears with local or systemic lymphadenopathy, e.g. infectious mononucleosis, toxoplasmosis, cat scratch disease, autoimmune diseases, sarcoidosis, tuberculotic lymphadenopathy and drug induced lymphadenopathy. Lymph node metastases of solid tumors and other non-Hodgkin's lymphomas (DLBCL, primary mediastinal B-cell lymphoma or T-cell/ histiocyte rich B-cell lymphoma) may also imply a difficult histopathological differential diagnostic problem. Complementary serology, immunohistochemistry, autoantibody assessment are needed.

PROGNOSTIC FACTORS

Early (I-II) Stage EORTC [38]

Presence of one factor results in unfavorable prognosis

- Age ≥ 50 years
- Number of affected region >3
- Bulky tumor
- Sedimentation rate > 50mm/h (no B-symptoms), or >30mm/h (B-symptoms)

Advanced Stage (III-IV) (IPS: International Prognostic Score) [39]

Every factor results one point, best prognosis: 0 point, worst: 7 points
Standard risk: 0-3 points, unfavorable: >3 points

- Age ≥ 45 years
- Male gender
- Stage IV.
- Albumin level < 40 g/L
- Hemoglobin < 105 g/L
- White blood cells > 15G/L

- Lymphocytes < 0.6 G/L or 8%

General condition (Eastern Cooperative Oncology Group (ECOG) performance status), co-morbidities and compliance of the patient should be also clarified.

^{18}Fluoro-Deoxy-Glucose Positron Emission Tomography/Computed Tomography

Recently ^{18}Fluoro-deoxy-glucose positron emission tomography/computed tomography (^{18}FDG PET/CT) is used for staging and restaging in HL. Response to treatment is evaluated based on the Cheson criteria. Complete remission (CR) is considered when disappearance of all signs of the disease can be observed. Partial remission (PR) is considered, when regression of measurable disease and no new sites can be observed. Stable disease (SD) is a failure to attain CR/PR or PD. In case of relapse or progressive disease a new lesion or more than 50% of increase of a previously involved site must be seen [40].PET/CT helps to identify those early dynamic metabolic changes, which show excellent correlation with response to treatment not only after the time of restaging, but during the whole treatment regime, as well. Interim PET/CT performed after 1-3 cycles of chemotherapy shows a better correlation with the prognosis of the disease, than the currently used conventional prognostic factors. However there is an ongoing debate, how response to treatment should be evaluated. Gallamini et al. first reported the superior prognostic value of interim PET/CT after 2 cycles of ABVD over IPS. PET/CT scans were interpreted visually and considered positive, negative or MRU (minimal residual uptake), which they considered as low-grade FDG uptake with avidity smaller than, equal to or only slightly higher than the uptake in mediastinal blood pool structures [41]. The International Harmonization Project suggests a 5-point scale, using liver and mediastinum, as reference organs [42]. Barrington et al. defined MRU as an uptake less than or equal to normal liver uptake [43]. Evaluating the early response to treatment gives a good chance to change treatment immediately.

Treating Hodgkin's Lymphoma

The goal of the treatment is always to cure the patient. Being a systemic disease, surgical procedure is not suitable, except for the lymph node biopsy. Current standard of care consists of polichemotherapy and radiotherapy. Currently irradiation is less used. Choosing treatment strategy is based on histological subtype, stage, prognostic factors, the patients' age, general condition and co-morbidities. Response to treatment should be evaluated in every 2 cycles during treatment. The degree and speed of response could be also a good prognostic factor. Treatment should be continued until significant regression can be seen; afterwards another 1-2 cycles should be administered.Definitive treatment group based on histological subtypes, stage and prognostic factors [33, 44-47].

I. Histology

Nodular lymphocyte predominant HL (NLPHL),

Classical HL (cHL)
Intermediate form between cHL and DLBCL

II. Stage and prognostic factors
Early favorable stage
Early unfavorable stage
Advanced standard stage
Advanced unfavorable stage

III. Age, co-morbidities, general conditions
Childhood HL
Elderly HL
HL in pregnancy
Patients with severe co-morbidities, which determines life expectancy
Patients, not treatable with chemotherapy

First Line Treatment of cHL

1. Early favorable HL (Figure 2,3)
    - 2-4 cycles ABVD (Adriamycin, Bleomycin, Vincristin, Dacarbazin) + IF-RT (30-35 Gy) (I/A evidence)
    - Chemotherapy alone (subject of current clinical trials)
    - EBVD (Epirubicin, Bleomycin, Vincristin, Dacarbazin) is also common, which is more beneficial regarding cardiological side effects, than ABVD
    - If anthracyclin is contraindicated, COPP (Cyclophosphamide, Vincristin, Procarbazine, Prednisone) regimen should be used

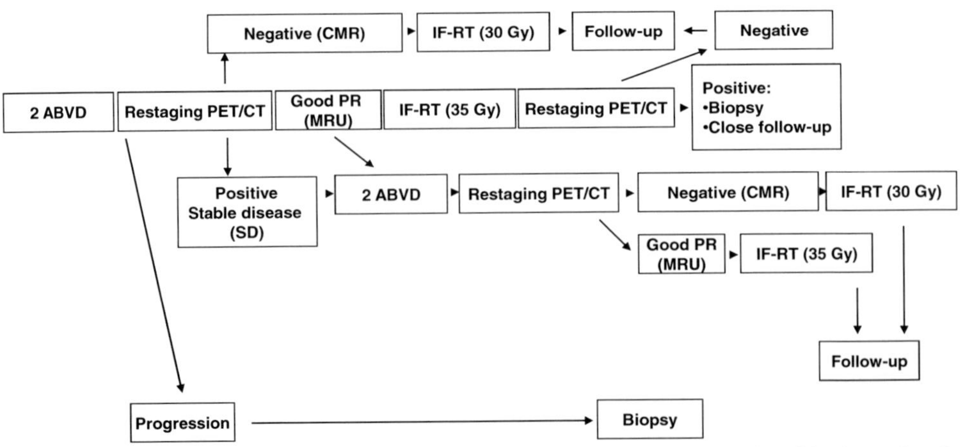

CMR - complete metabolic response, PR – partial response, MRU – minimal residual uptake, IF-RT - Involved field radiotherapy, ABVD - Adriamycin, Bleomycin, Vincristin, Dacarbazin, PET/CT - positron emission tomography computed tomography.

Figure 2. Treatment of early stage Hodgkin's lymphoma with favorable prognosis.

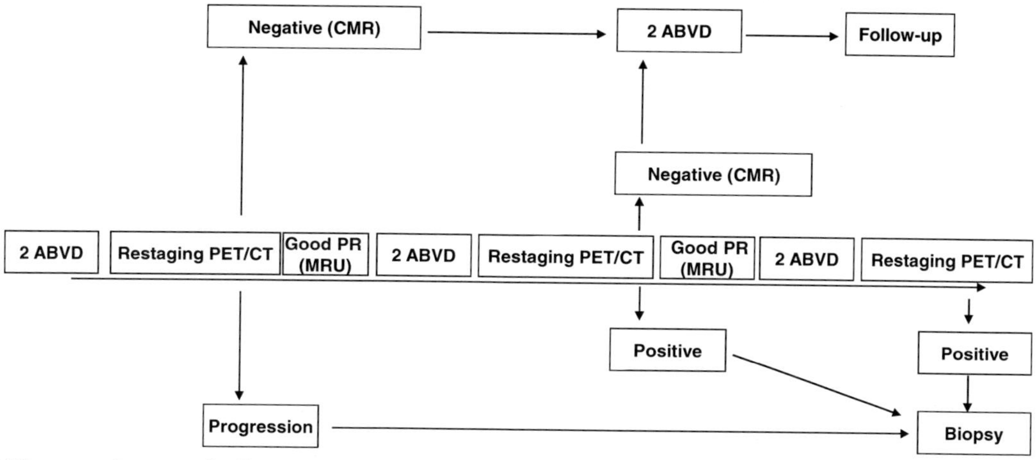

CMR - complete metabolic response, PR – partial response, MRU – minimal residual uptake, IF-RT - Involved field radiotherapy, ABVD - Adriamycin, Bleomycin, Vincristin, Dacarbazin, PET/CT - positron emission tomography computed tomography .

Figure 3. Treatment without irradiation of early stage Hodgkin's lymphoma with favorable prognosis.

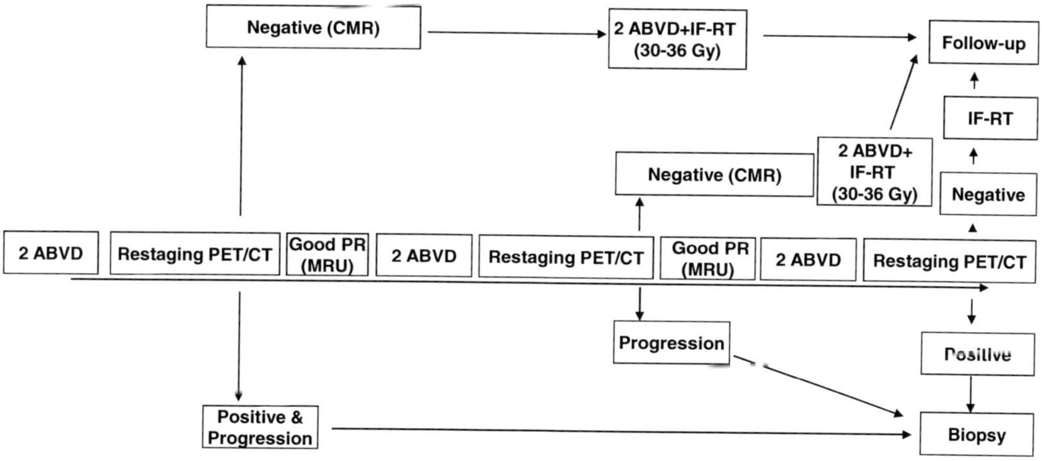

CMR - complete metabolic response, PR – partial response, MRU – minimal residual uptake, IF-RT - Involved field radiotherapy, ABVD - Adriamycin, Bleomycin, Vincristin, Dacarbazin, PET/CT - positron emission tomography computed tomography.

Figure 4. Treatment of early stage Hodgkin's lymphoma with unfavorable prognosis (bulky disease).

2. Early unfavorable HL (Figure 4)

- 4-6 cycles ABVD + IF-RT (30-35 Gy) (I/A evidence)

3. Advanced standard HL (Figure 5)

- 6-8 cycles ABVD (I/A evidence)
- Irradiation is only needed, when bulky or limited disease is present

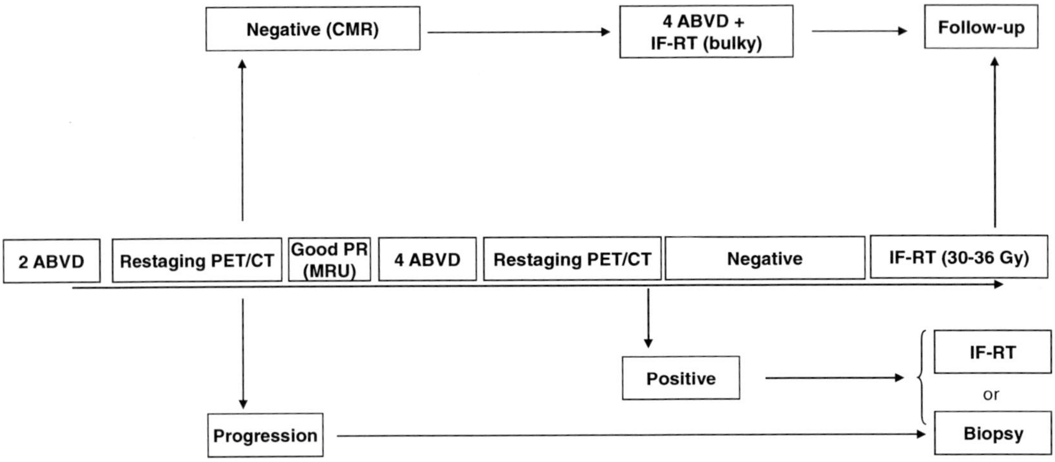

CMR - complete metabolic response, PR – partial response, MRU – minimal residual uptake, IF-RT - Involved field radiotherapy, ABVD - Adriamycin, Bleomycin, Vincristin, Dacarbazin, PET/CT - positron emission tomography computed tomography.

Figure 5. Treatment of advanced stage Hodgkin's lymphoma with standard prognosis.

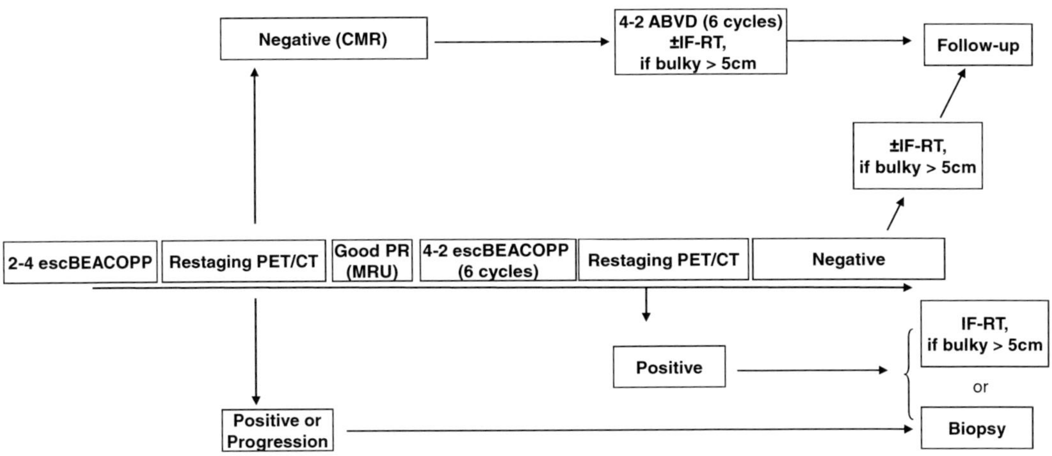

CMR - complete metabolic response, PR – partial response, MRU – minimal residual uptake, IF-RT - Involved field radiotherapy, ABVD - Adriamycin, Bleomycin, Vincristin, Dacarbazin, escBEACOPP - Bleomycin, Etoposid, Adriamycin, Cyclophosphamide, Vincristin, Procarbazin, Prednisolone escalated, PET/CT - positron emission tomography computed tomography.

Figure 6. Treatment of advanced stage Hodgkin's lymphoma with unfavorable prognosis.

4. Advanced unfavorable HL (Figure 6)

- 2-4 cycles BEACOPP escalated (Bleomycin, Etoposid, Adriamycin, Cyclophosphamide, Vincristin, Procarbazin, Prednisolone) followed by another 2-4 cycles of BEACOPP escalated or 4-2 cycles of ABVD (6 cycles in total) + involved field radiation (IF-RT) to affected regions measuring more than 5 cms.

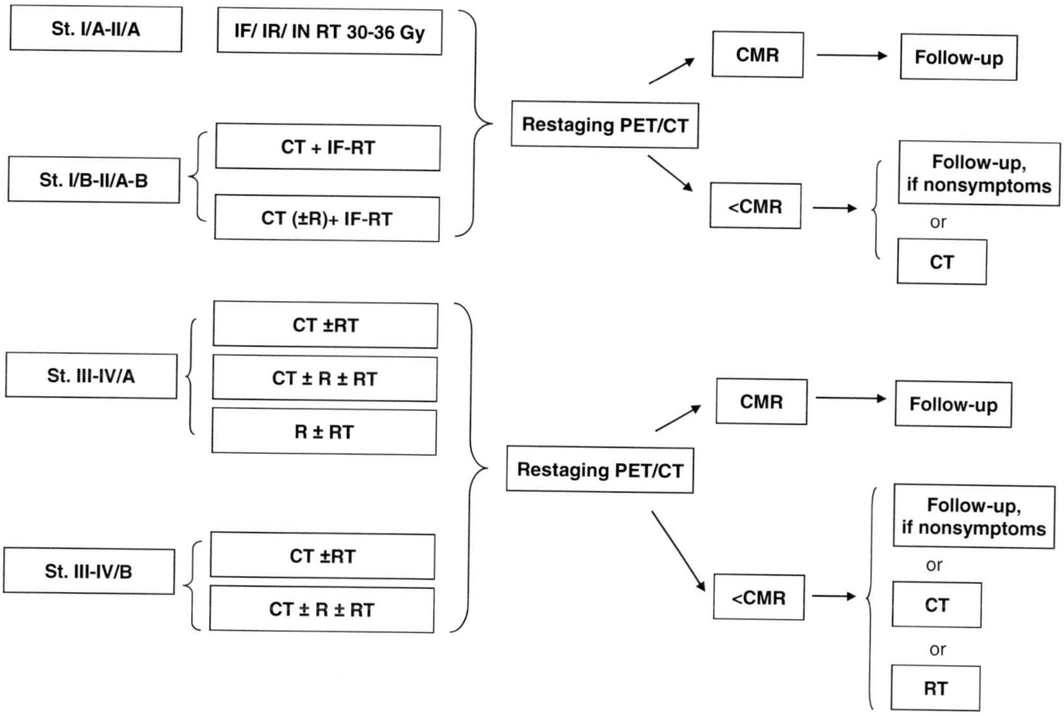

Figure 7. Treatment of nodular lymphocyte predominant Hodgkin's lymphoma.

IF-RT - Involved field, IR-RT - involved region, IN-RT - involved nodal radiotherapy, CMR - complete metabolic response, R – Rituximab.

First Line Treatment of NLPHL (Figure 7)

- "Watch and wait" strategy should be considered in cases of small tumor mass
- Stage I/A: Involved field (IF-RT), involved region (IR-RT), involved nodal (IN-RT) radiotherapy with 35 Gy of dose (in case of total excision 30Gy)
- Treatment of other cases are similar to other cHL (I/A evidence)
- Treatment of Advanced stage disease is similar to cHL (II/A evidence)
- Note: Based on CD20 expression, rituximab is considered to be beneficial, however it is not standard of care: rituximab-ABVD, 375 mg/m2 iv. on 1. and 15. days of cycle

Treatment of Other Subgroups

Elderly HL
Considering biological age and co-morbidities, treatment can be palliative or curative
Curative:

- Early favorable stage
    - only IF-RT
    - 2-4 cycles of A(E)BVD+IF-RT
    - 4 cycles CO(V)PP+IF-RT
- Early unfavorable stage, advanced stage
    - 4-6 cycles EBVD+-IF-RT
    - 6 cycles CO(V)PP+-IF-RT

Intermediate form between cHL and DLBCL

- Rituximab + chemotherapy (rituximab is on-label in this case)+IF-RT (considering an almost always present mediastinal bulky)
- Chemotherapy might be CHOP14 or 21 (alternatively dose adjusted EPOCH), considering the more aggressive disease
- Interim PET/CT should be performed after every 2 cycles
- In case of relapsed/refractory disease R-DHAP (rituximab, Dexamethason, Cytarabine, Cisplatin) or R-ICE (rituximab, ifosfamide, carboplatin, etoposide) salvage regimen, followed by high-dose chemo/radiotherapy (HDT) and autologous hematopoietic stem cell transplantation (AHSCT)

HL in pregnancy
First trimester
Early stage

- "Watch and Wait"
- IF/IN-RT in case of cervical involvement
- Abdominal defense in case of axillary involvement
- Vinblastin monotherapy
- Afterwards in second and third trimester ABVD can be given

Advanced stage

- Procure an abortion is suggested, followed by ABVD+-IF-RT

Second and third trimester
Early stage

- "Watch and Wait", treatment can be given after delivery

Advanced stage

- ABVD, delivery should be delayed to the non-cytopenic period

HL patients with severe co-morbidities

- Steroid
- Irradiation
- Reduced dose chemotherapy (CVPP, CHOP, ABVD), reduces number of cytostatics (CVP, AVD, ABV, VBM)

HL patients not treatable with chemotherapy

- Irradiation
- Early stage I/A - favorable - IFRT or EFRT (mantle or inverted Y)
- Early stage – other subgroups - EFRT (mantle, mantle+paraaortic, inverted Y)
- Advanced stage - EFRT, sTNI

Treatment of Primary Refractory/Relapsed HL

Change of therapy for patients with inadequate response to primary treatment depends on [33, 47]:

- Response to treatment (complete remission was not achieved, or patient was refractory to treatment (relapse after 6 months of therapy is also considered refractory)
- First line therapy
- General condition of the patient
- Expected outcome and risk (curative or palliative intent)

Treatment of patient relapsed after achieving complete remission after first line treatment depends on:

- Time spent in complete remission (CR) (the longer time spent in CR, the better is the prognosis)
- Localization of disease (localized, disseminated)
- Previous treatment, outcome

In case of relapse, the previously recommended investigation strategy is recommended, however another lymph node biopsy should be performed in case of relapse after one year.

General Considerations

- Chemotherapy after the irradiation can be used with same success rate as being primary treatment.
- Local relapse after chemotherapy, irradiation may be considered, however it is rarely sufficient.

- Relapse one year after the last chemotherapy, re-induction can be considered with first line chemotherapy, but another not cross-resistant chemotherapy can be used also
- Patients not responding adequately to first line treatment (stable) or primary refractory to chemotherapy (progressive) or relapse within 3 years after finishing chemotherapy, or who have repeated chemosensitive relapses observed up to three years after the chemotherapy, medium dose, salvage therapy (DHAP, ICE, IGEV, VIM, Dexa-BEAM, the mini-BEAM) should be given.
- If the patient is responsive, the patient should be prepared for high dose therapy and autologous hematopoietic stem cell transplantation, since results are better than the standard treatment
- More than 2-4 cycles of medium dose treatment is rarely used, response to treatment should be evaluated after every cycle
- NLPHL cases should be irradiated (IF-RT / IN-RT / IR-RT), in case of locally/ limited relapses, radiation therapy can be repeated as needed. Rituximab is an off-label alternative treatment.
- If high-dose therapy is unmet, another type of not cross-resistant chemotherapy can be chosen
- Second line chemotherapy options:

  - After ABVD - DHAP, ICE, IGEV, BEACOPP, CO (A) PP, CEP
  - After CO(V)PP - ABVD, BEACOPP, DHAP, ICE, IGEV

- Third line or further chemotherapy regimens, after high-dose therapy and AHSCT can be only chosen considering several criteria and can be determined individually. Participation in clinical trials can be recommended.
- Mortality of allergenic transplantation is very high (30-50%), if needed, reduced-intensity conditioning (RIC) can be tried, which has lower mortality.

Expected Side Effects, Prevention and Treating Complications

- In case of nausea and vomiting induced by cytotoxic agents, or irradiation, antiemetics (ondansetron, tropisetron, granisetron) should be given
- In case of severe pain, analgetics should be given
- Every antitumor therapy should be accompanied by inhibitors of uric acid synthesis (allopurinol)
- Proton pump inhibitors or H2-receptor antagonist should accompany steroid administration and / or antacid, furthermore potassium supplementation is required.
- In case of lytic bone lesions, bisphosphonate is recommended.
- In case of myelotoxicity due to treatment, anemia should be treated with transfusions (elected, filtered, irradiated), thrombocytopenia should be treated with platelet infusion. Febrile neutropenia should be treated as prophylaxis or intervention by myeloid colony stimulating factor (filgrastim, pegfilgrastim), furthermore appropriate antimicrobial therapy is indicated.

- For thrombosis prophylaxis low molecular weight heparin (LMWH) is recommended
- In case of severe alopecia due to chemotherapy wig should be ordered
- Emergency care may be needed in case of superior vena cava syndrome, tumor lysis syndrome, disseminated intravascular coagulation (DIC), ITP, AIHA.
- Due to nephrotoxicity of some cytostatic drugs increased rehydration is necessary.
- Vinca alkaloids (e.g. vincristin) causes neuropathy, anthracyclines causes cardiomyopathy, bleomycin causes pulmonary fibrosis and skin pigmentation, some cytostatic drugs cause sterility. After several years of administering alkylating cytostatic drugs secondary malignant hematological diseases, such as non-Hodgkin's lymphoma, myelodysplastic syndrome, acute myeloid leukemia may occur.
- Early radio-dermatitis may occur due to irradiation, after years and decades, secondary solid tumor, hypothyroidism, valvulopathy, pulmonary fibrosis and early coronary sclerosis may occur.

Control Tests Recommended During Treatment

- General condition, blood count, sera biochemical parameters should be checked before treatment.
- 7-10 days after the first treatment, blood count should be checked, whether transient cytopenia can be observed. If not 10-30% increase of dosage is recommended.
- In case of lower cell numbers before treatment, dose reduction and postponing treatment should be avoided, since reduction of dose intensity can significantly reduce outcome, thus colony stimulating factors should be administered
- After the second and fourth cycles of chemotherapy, general condition should be checked, which is recommended to measure the effectiveness and response to treatment (physical examination, abnormal laboratory and imaging tests before treatment requires interim PET / CT or CT)
- Special considerations for rehabilitation do not exist. The patient can work during treatment similar or minimal changes of life can be expected

Follow-Up of HL Patients

- After one month of completion of therapy, abnormal tests should be repeated
- 18FDG PET / CT shows unique benefits regarding evaluating response to treatment 6-8 weeks after completion of therapy. (Restaging PET/CT) Evaluation is performed based on the Cheson criteria [40].
- After achieving complete remission, patients' follow-up should be carried out due to the risk of relapse in every 1-2 months in the first year, every three months during the second-third year and every year-half year lifelong. Chest X-ray, abdominal and / or carotid ultrasound, physical examination and blood tests are recommended in every 2-3 months in the first year, in every 6 months in the second-third years, then annually.

- In case of partial remission, if no further treatment is performed, follow-up is recommended monthly in the first year then every two months in the second year. Performing 18FDG PET/ CT is only recommended in the reasonable suspicion of progression or relapse

If relapse is suspected the following investigations should be performed:

- If relapse occurs within one year: radiological progression, or cytology is acceptable, histology is not necessary.
- If relapse occurs over one year: repeated histological confirmation is necessary, cytology can be accepted only in exceptional cases
- In case of relapse, staging is recommended, described previously in order to evaluate the stage of the relapse

Eventually follow-up has to cover late complications of anticancer therapy.

In case of irradiation of the cervical region, thyroid hormone test is recommended annually, in case of chest-mediastinal irradiation, electrocardiography, ergometry, echocardiography, pulmonary function tests, breast ultrasound for women under 40 years of age, mammography for above 40 years of age need to be performed.

Future Treatment Strategies

Current combined modality treatment has its own cost, late side effects are remarkable, minimizing treatment toxicity is important, thus medicine is seeking for less intensive treatment protocols and targeted therapeutic approaches [48].

The German Hodgkin's Lymphoma Study Group showed, that 2 cycles of ABVD followed by 20 Gy IF-RT was as effective and less toxic as more intense combinations in early favorable stage HL [49], furthermore even dismissing irradiation may be possible in this patient population, while the overall survival was found to be better [50].

In early unfavorable stage HL, 2 cycles of escBEACOPP followed by 2 cycles of ABVD + 30 Gy IF-RT showed superiority compared to 4 cycles of ABVD followed by 30 Gy IF-RT, which has been considered as standard of care, so far [51]. Fewer relapses and late toxicities have been observed, however the frequency of acute toxicities was increased.

Less is considered more in advanced stage HL; 6 cycles of escBEACOPP followed by PET guided irradiation (30 Gy) was found to be equally efficient, however less toxic [52].

Brentuximab-vedotin (SGN-35), an antibody-drug conjugate (anti-CD30 antibody conjugated with monomethyl auristatin E) was approved by the US Food and Drug Administration for the treatment of CD30 positive relapsed/refractory lymphomas, HL and anaplastic large cell lymphoma in 2011 [53].

In the future, these promising compounds may be combined with current chemotherapy, thus improving patients' outcome. There is a new ongoing trial combining brentuximab vedotin with ABVD or AVD in the frontline setting [54]. The combination with AVD was associated with no significant pulmonary toxicity, while the one with ABVD showed significant toxicity.

Investigations on rituximab (anti-CD20 antibody) plus ABVD chemotherapy for advanced stage HL patients showed promising results, thus a large multicenter phase II clinical trial is currently enrolling patients [55].

The leading histone deacetylase inhibitor (HDACi) panobinostat (LBH589) has been involved in several clinical trials investigating relapsed/refractory HL patients, which shows promising results. The rationale of using these compounds is, that loss of B-cell phenotype of the HRS cells is epigenetically regulated, which might be therapeutically reversed [56].

The mechanistic target of rapamycin (mTOR) inhibitor, everolimus as single agent showed poor results [57], however it may be beneficial in combination with other compounds. Everolimus and panobinostat shows promising clinical activity in relapsed/refractory HL patients [58].

Recently lenalidomide was reported to show promising results in heavily pre-treated HL patients, results were comparable with panobinostat, however modest compared to brentuximab vedotin [59].

PROGNOSIS

Currently 80-85% of Hodgkin's lymphoma patients are expected to achieve complete remission with current first line treatment. Patients diagnosed in early stage are expected to have a 90% of 10-year disease-free survival (healing). Advanced stage standard risk patients are expected a 75-80% 10-year disease-free survival. Although advanced unfavorable stage patients have only a 70% of 10-year disease-free survival, due to excessive number of clinical trials further improvement is expected in this subgroup, as well. Primary chemo-resistant, refractory and relapsing patients after HDT + AHSCT have poor prognosis (80% die within one year).

The further characterization of the complex multi-step etiology and pathogenesis of Hodgkin's lymphoma will help in future drug developments, expectantly leading to increased remission rates and better survival in the disease.

REFERENCES

[1] Campo, E., Swerdlow, S.H., Harris, N.L., et al., The 2008 WHO classification of lymphoid neoplasms and beyond: evolving concepts and practical applications. *Blood,* 2011. *117*(19): p. 5019-5032.

[2] Thomas, R., Re, D., Wolf, J., and Diehl, V., Part I: Hodgkin's lymphoma--molecular biology of Hodgkin and Reed-Sternberg cells. *Lancet Oncol,* 2004. *5*(1): p. 11-18.

[3] Mack, T., Cozen, W., Shibata, D., et al., Concordance for Hodgkin's disease in identical twins suggesting genetic susceptibility to the young-adult form of the disease. *N. Engl. J. Med.,* 1995. *332*(7): p. 413-418.

[4] Straus, S.E., Jaffe, E.S., Puck, J.M., et al., The development of lymphomas in families with autoimmune lymphoproliferative syndrome with germline Fas mutations and defective lymphocyte apoptosis. *Blood,* 2001. *98*(1): p. 194-200.

[5] Jarrett, R.F., Viruses and Hodgkin's lymphoma. *Ann. Onc.,* 2002. *13*(suppl_1): p. 23-29.

[6] Re, D., Kuppers, R., and Diehl, V., Molecular Pathogenesis of Hodgkin's Lymphoma. *J. Clin. Oncol.,* 2005. *23*(26): p. 6379-6386.

[7] Pileri, S.A., Ascani, S., Leoncini, L., et al., Hodgkin's lymphoma: the pathologist's viewpoint. *J. Clin. Pathol.,* 2002. *55*(3): p. 162-176.

[8] Stein, H., Marafioti, T., Foss, H.-D., et al., Down-regulation of BOB.1/OBF.1 and Oct2 in classical Hodgkin disease but not in lymphocyte predominant Hodgkin disease correlates with immunoglobulin transcription. *Blood,* 2001. *97*(2): p. 496-501.

[9] Busslinger, M., Transcriptional control of early B cell development. *Annu. Rev. Immunol.,* 2004. *22*: p. 55-79.

[10] Mathas, S., Janz, M., Hummel, F., et al., Intrinsic inhibition of transcription factor E2A by HLH proteins ABF-1 and Id2 mediates reprogramming of neoplastic B cells in Hodgkin lymphoma. *Nat. Immunol.,* 2006. *7*(2): p. 207-215.

[11] Jundt, F., Anagnostopoulos, I., Forster, R., et al., Activated Notch1 signaling promotes tumor cell proliferation and survival in Hodgkin and anaplastic large cell lymphoma. *Blood,* 2002. *99*(9): p. 3398-3403.

[12] Mathas, S., The pathogenesis of classical Hodgkin's lymphoma: a model for B-cell plasticity. *Hematol. Oncol. Clin. North. Am.,* 2007. *21*(5): p. 787-804.

[13] Mathas, S., Lietz, A., Anagnostopoulos, I., et al., c-FLIP Mediates Resistance of Hodgkin/Reed-Sternberg Cells to Death Receptor-induced Apoptosis. *J. Exp. Med.,* 2004. *199*(8): p. 1041-1052.

[14] Kashkar, H., Haefs, C., Shin, H., et al., XIAP-mediated Caspase Inhibition in Hodgkin's Lymphoma-derived B Cells. *J. Exp. Med.,* 2003. *198*(2): p. 341-347.

[15] Tan, T. and Coussens, L., Humoral immunity, inflammation and cancer. *Curr. Opin. Immunol.,* 2007. *19*(2): p. 209-216.

[16] Poppema, S., Immunobiology and Pathophysiology of Hodgkin Lymphomas. ASH Education Program Book, 2005. *2005*(1): p. 231-238.

[17] Aldinucci, D., Gloghini, A., Pinto, A., De Filippi, R., and Carbone, A., The classical Hodgkin's lymphoma microenvironment and its role in promoting tumour growth and immune escape. *J. Pathol.,* 2010. *221*(3): p. 248-263.

[18] Gaidano, G., Hauptschein, R., Parsa, N., et al., Deletions involving two distinct regions of 6q in B-cell non-Hodgkin lymphoma. *Blood,* 1992. *80*(7): p. 1781-1787.

[19] Joos, S., Kupper, M., Ohl, S., et al., Genomic Imbalances Including Amplification of the Tyrosine Kinase Gene JAK2 in CD30+ Hodgkin Cells. *Cancer Res.,* 2000. *60*(3): p. 549-552.

[20] Kupper, M., Joos, S., von Bonin, F., et al., MDM2 gene amplification and lack of p53 point mutations in Hodgkin and Reed-Sternberg cells: results from single-cell polymerase chain reaction and molecular cytogenetic studies. *Br. J. Haematol.,* 2001. *112*(3): p. 768-775.

[21] Joos, S., Menz, C.K., Wrobel, G., et al., Classical Hodgkin lymphoma is characterized by recurrent copy number gains of the short arm of chromosome 2. *Blood,* 2002. *99*(4): p. 1381-1387.

[22] Martin-Subero, J.I., Gesk, S., Harder, L., et al., Recurrent involvement of the REL and BCL11A loci in classical Hodgkin lymphoma. *Blood,* 2002. *99*(4): p. 1474-1477.

[23] Steidl, C., Telenius, A., Shah, S.P., et al., Genome-wide copy number analysis of Hodgkin Reed-Sternberg cells identifies recurrent imbalances with correlations to treatment outcome. *Blood,* 2010. *116*(3): p. 418-427.

[24] Kuppers, R., Klein, U., Schwering, I., et al., Identification of Hodgkin and Reed-Sternberg cell-specific genes by gene expression profiling. *J. Clin. Invest.,* 2003. *111*(4): p. 529-537.
[25] Parkin, D. and Muir, C., Cancer Incidence in Five Continents. Comparability and quality of data. *IARC Sci. Publ.,* 1992(120): p. 45-173.
[26] Jemal, A., Siegel, R., Ward, E., et al., Cancer statistics, 2009. CA *Cancer J. Clin.,* 2009. *59*(4): p. 225-249.
[27] Siegel, R., Naishadham, D., and Jemal, A., Cancer statistics, 2012. CA *Cancer J. Clin.,* 2012. *62*(1): p. 10-29.
[28] Nogova, L., Rudiger, T., and Engert, A., Biology, Clinical Course and Management of Nodular Lymphocyte-Predominant Hodgkin Lymphoma. *Hematology,* 2006. *2006*(1): p. 266-272.
[29] Correa, P. and O'Conor, G., Epidemiologic patterns of Hodgkin's disease. *Int. J. Cancer,* 1971. *8*(2): p. 192-201.
[30] Eberle, F., Mani, H., and Jaffe, E., Histopathology of Hodgkin's lymphoma. *Cancer J.,* 2009. *15*(2): p. 129-137.
[31] Ansell, S. and Armitage, J., Management of Hodgkin lymphoma. *Mayo. Clin. Proc.,* 2006. *81*(3): p. 419-426.
[32] Engert, A., Eichenauer, D.A., Dreyling, M., and Group, O.b.o.t.E.G.W., Hodgkin's lymphoma: ESMO Clinical Recommendations for diagnosis, treatment and follow-up. *Annals of Oncology,* 2009. *20*(suppl 4): p. iv108-iv109.
[33] Illés, Á. and Molnár, Z., A felnőttkori Hodgkin-lymphoma ellátásának irányelvei, in Hematológiai betegségek korszerű kezelése, D. Lehocky, Editor. 2011. p. 285-309.
[34] Carbone, P.P., Kaplan, H.S., Musshoff, K., Smithers, D.W., and Tubiana, M., Report of the Committee on Hodgkin's Disease Staging Classification. *Cancer Research,* 1971. *31*(11): p. 1860-1861.
[35] Lister, T.A., Crowther, D., Sutcliffe, S.B., et al., Report of a committee convened to discuss the evaluation and staging of patients with Hodgkin's disease: Cotswolds meeting. *Journal of Clinical Oncology,* 1989. *7*(11): p. 1630-1636.
[36] Gallamini, A., Hutchings, M., Rigacci, L., et al., Early Interim 2-[18F]Fluoro-2-Deoxy-D-Glucose Positron Emission Tomography Is Prognostically Superior to International Prognostic Score in Advanced-Stage Hodgkin's Lymphoma: A Report From a Joint Italian-Danish Study. *Journal of Clinical Oncology,* 2007. *25*(24): p. 3746-3752.
[37] van der Kaaij, M.A.E., van Echten-Arends, J., Simons, A.H.M., and Kluin-Nelemans, H.C., Fertility preservation after chemotherapy for Hodgkin lymphoma. *Hematological Oncology,* 2010. *28*(4): p. 168-179.
[38] Tubiana, M., Henry-Amar, M., Carde, P., et al., Toward comprehensive management tailored to prognostic factors of patients with clinical stages I and II in Hodgkin's disease. The EORTC Lymphoma Group controlled clinical trials: 1964-1987. *Blood,* 1989. *73*(1): p. 47-56.
[39] Hasenclever, D. and Diehl, V., A prognostic score for advanced Hodgkin's disease. International Prognostic Factors Project on Advanced Hodgkin's Disease. *N. Engl. J. Med.,* 1998. *339*(21): p. 1506-1514.
[40] Cheson, B.D., Pfistner, B., Juweid, M.E., et al., Revised Response Criteria for Malignant Lymphoma. *Journal of Clinical Oncology,* 2007. *25*(5): p. 579-586.

[41] Gallamini, A., Hutchings, M., Rigacci, L., et al., Early Interim 2-[18F]Fluoro-2-Deoxy-D-Glucose Positron Emission Tomography Is Prognostically Superior to International Prognostic Score in Advanced-Stage Hodgkin's Lymphoma: A Report From a Joint Italian-Danish Study. *J. Clin. Oncol.,* 2007. *25*(24): p. 3746-3752.
[42] Meignan, M., Gallamini, A., and Haioun, C., Report on the First International Workshop on Interim-PET-Scan in Lymphoma. *Leuk Lymphoma,* 2009. *50*(8): p. 1257-1260.
[43] Barrington, S., Qian, W., Somer, E., et al., Concordance between four European centres of PET reporting criteria designed for use in multicentre trials in Hodgkin lymphoma. *Eur. J. Nucl. Med. Mol. Imaging.,* 2010. *37*(10): p. 1824-1833.
[44] Bartlett, N., Modern treatment of Hodgkin lymphoma. *Curr. Opin. Hematol.,* 2008. *15*(4): p. 408-414.
[45] Diehl, V., Thomas, R., and Re, D., Part II: Hodgkin's lymphoma--diagnosis and treatment. *Lancet Oncol.,* 2004. *5*(1): p. 19-26.
[46] NCCN Clinical Practice Guidelines in Oncology: *Hodgkin Lymphoma,* (version V.2.2012).
[47] Moskowitz, C., An update on the management of relapsed and primary refractory Hodgkin's disease. *Semin. Oncol.,* 2004. *31*(2 Suppl 4): p. 54-59.
[48] Jona, A. and Younes, A., Novel treatment strategies for patients with relapsed classical Hodgkin lymphoma. *Blood Reviews,* 2010. *24*(6): p. 233-238.
[49] Engert, A., Plutschow, A., Eich, H., et al., Reduced treatment intensity in patients with early-stage Hodgkin's lymphoma. *N. Engl. J. Med.,* 2010. *363*(7): p. 640-652.
[50] Meyer, R., Gospodarowicz, M., Connors, J., et al., ABVD alone versus radiation-based therapy in limited-stage Hodgkin's lymphoma. *N. Engl. J. Med.,* 2012. *366*(5): p. 399-408.
[51] von Tresckow, B., Plutschow, A., Fuchs, M., et al., Dose-Intensification in Early Unfavorable Hodgkin's Lymphoma: Final Analysis of the German Hodgkin Study Group HD14 Trial. *J. Clin. Oncol.,* 2012. *30*(9): p. 907-913.
[52] Engert, A., Haverkamp, H., Kobe, C., et al., Reduced-intensity chemotherapy and PET-guided radiotherapy in patients with advanced stage Hodgkin's lymphoma (HD15 trial): a randomised, open-label, phase 3 non-inferiority trial. *Lancet,* 2012.
[53] Younes, A., Bartlett, N.L., Leonard, J.P., et al., Brentuximab Vedotin (SGN-35) for Relapsed CD30-Positive Lymphomas. *New England Journal of Medicine,* 2010. *363*(19): p. 1812-1821.
[54] Younes, A., Connors, J.M., Park, S.I., Hunder, N.N.H., and Ansell, S.M., Frontline Therapy with Brentuximab Vedotin Combined with ABVD or AVD in Patients with Newly Diagnosed Advanced Stage Hodgkin Lymphoma. ASH *Annual Meeting Abstracts,* 2011. *118*(21): p. 955-.
[55] Younes, A., Oki, Y., McLaughlin, P., et al., Phase II study of rituximab plus ABVD in patients with newly diagnosed classical Hodgkin lymphoma. *Blood,* 2012.
[56] Sureda, A., Younes, A., Ben-Yehuda, D., et al., Final Analysis: Phase II Study of Oral Panobinostat In Relapsed/Refractory Hodgkin Lymphoma Patients Following Autologous Hematopoietic Stem Cell Transplant. *ASH Annual Meeting Abstracts,* 2010. *116*(21): p. 419-.
[57] Johnston, P., Inwards, D., Colgan, J., et al., A Phase II trial of the oral mTOR inhibitor everolimus in relapsed Hodgkin lymphoma. *Am. J. Hematol,* 2010. *85*(5): p. 320-324.

[58] Younes, A., Copeland, A., Fanale, M.A., et al., Safety and Efficacy of the Novel Combination of Panobinostat (LBH589) and Everolimus (RAD001) in Relapsed/Refractory Hodgkin and Non-Hodgkin Lymphoma. *ASH Annual Meeting Abstracts,* 2011. *118*(21): p. 3718-.
[59] Fehniger, T.A., Larson, S., Trinkaus, K., et al., A phase 2 multicenter study of lenalidomide in relapsed or refractory classical Hodgkin lymphoma. *Blood,* 2011. *118*(19): p. 5119-5125.

In: Hodgkin's and T-Cell Lymphoma
Editors: Warren K. Harvey and Randall M. Jacobs
ISBN 978-1-62257-478-0

Chapter 5

HIV-ASSOCIATED T-CELL LYMPHOMA: EPIDEMIOLOGY, PATHOBIOLOGY, CLINICAL FEATURES, PROGNOSIS AND MANAGEMENT

Prakash Vishnu[1] and David M. Aboulafia[2,*]
[1]Floyd and Delores Jones Cancer Institute
at Virginia Mason Medical Center, Seattle, WA, US
[2]Division of Hematology, University of Washington, Seattle, WA, US

ABSTRACT

T-*c*ell *l*ymphoma (TCL) occurrence in the setting of the *a*cquired *i*mmune *d*eficiency *s*yndrome (AIDS) and human immunodeficiency virus (HIV) infection is infrequent. The vast majority of *A*IDS-*r*elated *l*ymphomas (ARL) are of B-cell origin with TCL accounting for only 1.5-3% of all cases. Epidemiologic studies, however, suggest that people living with HIV/AIDS have a 15-fold higher risk of TCL compared to comparably matched but HIV-negative cohorts. While a direct causal role for HIV in T-cell lymphomagenesis is not established, co-infection with other oncogenic viruses including Epstein-Barr virus, hepatitis-C virus, and human T-lymphotropic virus type-I have been implicated in AIDS-related TCL (ARTCL). The diversity of viral co-infections linked to the various ARTCLs is illustrative of the histopathologic and clinical heterogeneity of these various non-Hodgkin's lymphomas. Although aggressive TCL portends a poor prognosis, several novel therapies have recently been shown to have significant activity in TCL. Whether these agents can be safely used in patients with ARTCL and with similar efficacy is a question of immediate clinical relevance.

INTRODUCTION

Lymphoma has been associated with *h*uman *i*mmunodeficiency *v*irus (HIV) infection since the beginning of the *a*cquired *i*mmune *d*eficiency *s*yndrome (AIDS) epidemic. In 1983

* Address correspondence to: David M. Aboulafia, MD: Telephone: (206) 341-1284 Fax: (206) 223-6914.

the *C*enter for *D*isease *C*ontrol and Prevention (CDC) included certain types of high-grade lymphomas in the catalog of AIDS-defining clinical conditions. [1] Prior to the advent of *h*ighly *a*ctive *a*nti-*r*etroviral *t*herapy (HAART) in 1996, *A*IDS-*r*elated *l*ymphomas (ARLs) were associated with a dismal prognosis, particularly in those patients who had compromised performance status, advanced immune dysfunction and limited hematopoietic reserve. With the introduction of HAART, the survival of these individuals is now comparable to their stage and histology matched HIV-negative lymphoma counterparts.

ARLs are primarily comprised of aggressive lymphomas of B-cell origin. However, epidemiological data from AIDS registries have linked HIV-infection with an increased risk of *T*-*c*ell *l*ymphoma (TCL). In contrast to B-cell ARL, ARTCLs have been reported less frequently. They are comprised of a heterogeneous and biologically diverse group of lymphomas that have been associated with a poor prognosis. Absent the introduction of a monoclonal antibody with synergistic activity with chemotherapy, along the lines of success of the anti-CD 20 monoclonal antibody Rituxan in *B*-*c*ell *l*ymphoma (BCL), treatment of TCLs have lagged behind that of aggressive BCL. The emergence of novel chemotherapy drugs with significant activity have, however, led to a renaissance in interest in the biology, clinical course and treatment options for these rare T-cell neoplasms.

EPIDEMIOLOGY

According to United States Surveillance Epidemiology and End Results data for the years 2005-2009, mature T- and Natural Killer (NK-) cell lymphomas are infrequent neoplasms with an age adjusted incidence rate of only 1.77/100,000 per year. [2] In the United States (US), they account for 10-12% of all lymphoid malignancies. [3]

The risk of TCL in people living with HIV/AIDS (PLWHA) is greater than in the general population. [3, 4] Unlike B-cell ARLs, current understanding of the incidence and spectrum of TCLs that occur in PLWA is rudimentary. Most available epidemiological data are retrospective and potentially underpowered, partly confounded by the difficulty in diagnosing and classifying this group of lymphomas. [5-8] Consequently, most quoted estimates of ARTCLs are derived from a single data set.

In 2001, investigators linked AIDS and cancer registry data from 1978 through 1996 in 11 state or metropolitan areas of the US. Overall, 366,034 AIDS patients were linked to local area cancer records and 6,788 cases of ARL were identified. of which 96 (1.4%) cases were of T-cell origin. [7] The estimated *r*elative *r*isk (RR) of TCL in the 2-year period after AIDS onset was 15 (95% CI: 10-21.7) with a statistically significant increase seen for all specific T-cell subtypes, varying from 8-fold for mycosis fungoides/Sézary syndrome to 24.4-fold for cutaneous lymphomas. The observed and expected incidence and RR of various subtypes of ARTCL are shown in Table 1. The RR of ARTCL was higher in Hispanics (RR 24.0, 95% CI: 8.8-52.3, n=6) than in Caucasian (RR 14.4, 95% CI: 6.9-26.6, n=10) or African-American patients (10.0, 95% CI: 4.6-19.1, n=9), although the incidence in persons with AIDS comparable by race/ethnicity (10.3, 7.0 and 8.7 per 100,000 person-years, respectively).

In a retrospective and single institution review of 429 consecutive HIV-infected patients diagnosed with ARLs, 11 (3%) were of T-cell origin consistent with data reported from the AIDS Cancer Match Registry. [5]

Table 1. Incidence and relative risk of AIDS-related T-cell lymphoma in the 2-year period after AIDS onset

	No. of cases		Incidence†		RR	95% CI
	O *	E **	O *	E **		
T-cell lymphomas	28	1.87	9.22	0.61	15	10.0-21.7
Mycosis fungoides/Sezary	8	1.01	2.59	0.33	8	3.4-15.7
Peripheral lymphoma	10	0.41	3.24	0.13	24.3	11.7-44.8
Cutaneous lymphoma	7	0.29	2.27	0.09	24.4	9.8-50.3
Adult T-cell leukemia/lymphoma	2	0.14	0.65	0.04	14.6	1.8-52.8
Angiocentric T-cell lymphoma	1	0.03	0.32	0.01	35.9	0.9-200.0
All non-Hodgkin's lymphoma	3,405	47	1,104.30	15.2	72.4	70.0-74.9

† per 100,000 person-years, * observed, ** expected.

Adapted from Biggar RJ, Engles EA, et al. Risk of T-Cell lymphoma in persons with AIDS. AIDS Cancer Match Registry Study Group. *JAIDS* 2001; 26(4):371.

Many of these patients were diagnosed in the pre-HAART era or shortly after HAART became widely available. Histopathologic subtypes included peripheral T-cell lymphoma in five; anaplastic large T-cell lymphoma (ALTCL) in three and angioimmunoblastic T-cell lymphoma (AITL), enteropathy type, and Human T-cell lymphotropic virus type-I (HTLV-I) related adult T-cell lymphoma/leukemia (ATLL) in one case each.

Recognizing the predilection of various TCLs to occur in higher incidence in certain geographic location, such as ATLL in Southern Japan and NK-cell lymphomas of the nasal type in Asia, further studies involving larger data sets from various countries are needed to obtain a more accurate perspective on the epidemiology of ARTCLs in the HAART era.

ETIOLOGY AND PATHOGENESIS

Infection with HIV is associated with a myriad of immunologic aberrations, but the mechanisms which promote lymphoma in the setting of HIV infection are not fully understood. [9] (Figure 1) Current evidence suggests that HIV contributes indirectly to lymphomagenesis, principally through immunological derangements and chronic antigenic stimulation. Oncoviruses (e.g., *E*pstein *B*arr *V*irus [EBV], HTLV-1, and *H*uman *H*erpes *V*irus Type-8 [HHV-8]) are associated with approximately half of systemic ARLs, indicating that viral oncogenes may also play an important role in lymphomagenesis. [10]HIV infection creates a milieu of combined immune suppression and chronic antigenic stimulation which can promote polyclonal, oligoclonal, and ultimately monoclonal B-cell populations. This environment with dysregulated cytokine release and impaired dendritic function, along with presence of concomitant viral infections, promotes a permissive environment for HIV-induced impaired T-cell immunosurveillance which can culminate in various lymphoproliferative disorders.

Disruption of the cytokine network and high serum levels of interleukin (IL)-6 and IL-10 are features of ARLs associated with EBV and HHV-8 co-infection. IL-6 is an autocrine growth factor in lymphoma, and HIV may further stimulate monocyte and macrophage production of IL-6. [11]

EBV is the prototypical DNA oncovirus associated with several lymphoproliferative disorders. Peripheral TCL subtypes such AITL and NK-TCL are tightly linked with EBV infection. [12] The precise role of EBV in T-lymphomagenesis is not completely understood but appears to be related to selective immunosuppression and cytokine dysregulation via B- and T-cells.

Approximately 90% of primary effusion lymphomas (PELs) are associated with HHV-8 and 30% are associated with EBV co-infection. These rare tumors have a predilection to migrate to serous compartments including the pleura and pericardium and are generally poorly responsive to chemotherapy. Often, they are of null lymphocyte immunophenotype and occasionally associated with markers of plasmacytic differentiation; rarely PELs are associated with a T-cell phenotype and with HHV-8 infection. [13] There is growing evidence that HHV-8 is directly lymphomagenic. HHV-8 encoded products, such as latent associated nuclear antigen1 and viral IL-6 that inactivate p53 transcriptional activity, cause chemokine derangements and promote angiogenesis. [14]

HTLV-1 and HTLV-II co-infection have also been reported in patients with ARTCL, and in a few of these cases, the viral genome is present in the neoplastic cells. One may suspect HTLV-I and HIV co-infection in the correct clinical context and when the patient is experiencing classic AIDS-defining opportunistic infections such as oral thrush, Pnuemocysis Carinii pneumonia, and Cytomegalovirus retinitis despite well preserved CD4+ cell counts. [15]

Shortly after the widespread adoption of HAART in 1996 there occurred a significant decrease in the incidence of ARL. [16] Data from the Swiss HIV cohort study, which included 12,959 PLWHA, showed that between the years 1993 to 1995 the incidence of lymphoma was 13.6 per 100,000 person-years, and this declined to 1.8 per 100,000 in the period between 2002 and 2006. [17]

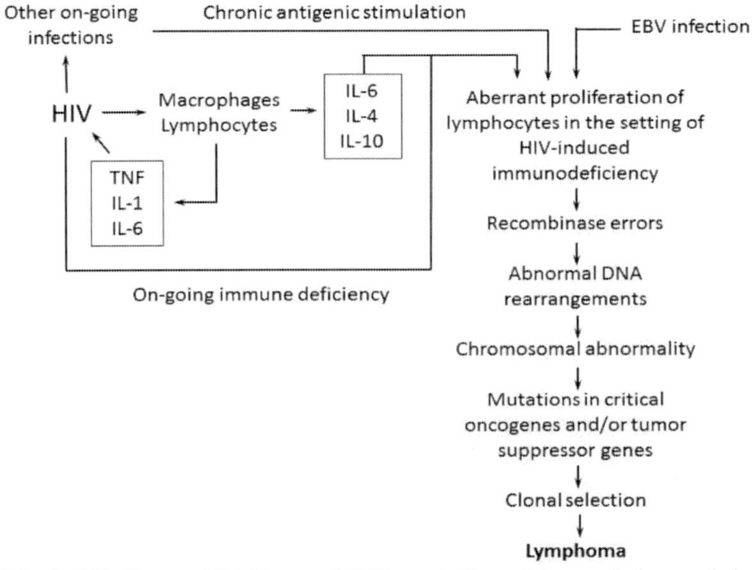

Modified from Martin JN, Ganem DE, Osmond DH, et al. Sexual transmission and the natural history of human herpes virus 8 infection. *N. Eng. J. Med.* 338:948, 1998.

Figure 1. Schematic representation of possible events resulting in development of lymphoma in patients with HIV.

HAART may also modify T-cell lymphomagenic stimuli in several ways, such as improving responsiveness of EBV-specific cytotoxic T-cell lymphocytes, increasing EBV-specific antibodies, and stabilizing immune perturbations that may contribute to T-cell proliferation.

Pathology and Immunophenotypic Features

The WHO Classification of lymphoid malignancies divides those associated with HIV infection into three categories: (1) lymphomas also occurring in immunocompetent patients, including TCL; (2) lymphoma occurring more specifically in HIV-positive patients, like PEL of T-cell immunophenotype; and (3) lymphoma occurring in other immunodeficiency states. [18] (Table 2)

Table 2. WHO Classification of lymphoid malignancies associated with HIV infection

Lymphomas also occurring in immunocompetent patients
Burkitt and Burkitt-like lymphomas
Diffuse large B-cell lymphomas
- Centroblastic
- Immunoblastic (including primary CNS lymphoma)
Extranodal MALT lymphoma (rare)
Peripheral T-cell lymphoma (rare)
Classical Hodgkin lymphoma
Lymphoma occurring more specifically in HIV-positive patients
Primary effusion lymphoma
Plasmablastic lymphoma of the oral cavity
Lymphoma occurring in other immunodeficiency states
Polymorphic B-cell lymphoma (PTLD-like) (rare)

MALT: marginal zone lymphoma of mucosa-associated lymphoid tissue;
PTLD: post transplant lymphoproliferative disorder; CNS: central nervous system.
Source: Swerdlow, SH, Campo, E, Harris, NL, et al. (Eds). World Health Organization Classification of Tumours of Haematopoietic and Lymphoid Tissues. IARC Press: Lyon 2008.

Table 3. Subtypes of published AIDS-related T-cell lymphoma

T-cell lymphoma subtype	Number of cases	Percentage
PTCL-unspecified (PTCL-U)	36	42
Anaplastic large cell lymphoma (ALCL)	24	28
NK/T-cell lymphoma	6	7
T-cell primary CNS lymphoma	6	7
Adult T-cell leukemia/lymphoma (ATLL)	4	5
Angioimmunoblastic T-cell lymphoma (AITL)	4	5
T-cell primary effusion lymphoma (PEL)	3	4
Enteropathy-like T-cell lymphoma (ELTL)	1	1
Subcutaneous panniculitis like T-cell lymphoma (SPTCL)	1	1

Adapted from Castillo JJ, Perez K, et al. Peripheral T-cell lymphomas in HIV-infected individuals: a comprehensive review. *J. HIV Therapy*.2009; 14(2):34-40.

Table 4. Selected pathologic characteristics of AIDS-related T-cell lymphoma

Lymphoma subtype	Number of cases	ALK tested	ALK positive	EBER tested	EBER positive	Ki67 tested	Ki67 positive	TCR tested	TCR positive
PTCL-U	31	7	0 (0%)	10	3 (30%)	9	5 (56%)	8	4 (50%)
ALCL	11	7	0 (0%)	2	1 (50%)	0	NA	5	3 (60%)
NK/TCL	7	2	0 (0%)	6	4 (67%)	3	1 (33%)	2	1 (50%)
AITL	2	2	0 (0%)	2	0 (0%)	2	0 (0%)	1	1 (100%)
Total	51	18	0 (0%)	20	8 (40%)	14	6 (43%)	16	9 (56%)

PTCL-U: PTCL-unspecified; ALCL: Anaplastic large cell lymphoma; NK/TCL: NK/T-cell lymphoma; AITL: Angioimmunoblastic T-cell lymphoma.

Adapted from Castillo JJ, Beltran BE, et al. Prognostic factors in pateints with HIV-associated peripheral T-cell lymphoma: A multicenter study. *Am. J. Hematol.* 2011; 86:256.

A wide spectrum of TCLs in PLWHA exists, including mycosis fungoides/Sézary syndrome, cutaneous TCL, peripheral TCL- unspecified (PTCL-U), ALTCL, NK-TCL, T-cell primary CNS lymphoma (PCNSL), HTLV-I -associated ATLL, AITL, T-cell PEL and enteropathy-like TCL (ELTL). [5-8, 13] (Table 3) In an international multicenter study of 51 cases of HIV-associated PTCL, PTCL-unspecified was the most common sub-type (n=31, 61%), followed by ALCL (n=11, 22%), NK-TCL (n=7, 14%) and AITL (n=2, 4%). [6] Select pathologic characteristics of these cases are shown in Table 4.

The immunophenotypic designation of TCL is based on the expression of at least one pan-T antigen and/or one subset T-antigen, and no pan-B antigen expression. [8] The commonly expressed T-cell antigens include CD45RO, CD43, CD3, CD4, CD5 and CD8. CD56 is expressed in NK-TCL. ALCL has a highly pleomorphic appearance, including the hallmark ‘anaplastic’ cells and exhibit uniform expression of CD30 (Ki-1). Unlike ALCL in immune competent patients, AIDS-related ALCL is reported to have very low expression of ALK-1 (0-11%) by immunohistochemistry and no detectable ALK gene rearrangement abnormalities. T-cell receptor gene rearrangement by polymerase chain reaction (PCR) is demonstrable in most cases of ARTCL. Average expression of Ki-67, a nuclear antigen protein which is used to determine the growth fraction of tumors, is 60% with a range of 10-95%. [5, 6, 13] In an international multicenter study of HIV-associated PTCL, PTCL-U, NK-TCL and AITL had an average expression of Ki-67 of 75%, 0% and 25%, respectively. [6]

Morphologic features of AITL include prominent vascularization of arborizing venules, expansion of follicular dendritic cell networks, and identification of CD10 as a phenotypic marker of neoplastic cells. HTLV-1-associated ATTL frequently contains neoplastic cells with a distinct cloverleaf appearance. Of note, aggressive AIDS-related BCLs occasionally lack CD20 and exhibit aberrant T-cell antigen expression, which may falsely lead to an impression of TCL. [19] As such, all pathology specimens should be reviewed in a Pathology Center that has broad experience interpreting HIV/AIDS-associated lymphoproliferations.

Clinical Features

ARTCL has primarily been reported in young adults with a median age at diagnosis of 38 years (range, 16-66 years); 99% of these cases have involved individuals less than 60 years of age. [5, 6, 13] The male to female ratio is 4:1. [6, 13] These age and gender associations are expected to change as the life expectancy of PLWHA continues to improve and a disproportionately increased number of women become HIV infected. Among Western countries with ready access to HAART the median age of PLWHA is now 50 years old. [20]

According to data from the AIDS Cancer Match Registry, the incidence of ARTCL is 10.3, 7.0, and 8.7 per 100,000 person-years among Hispanics, Caucasians and African-Americans, respectively. [7] This suggests similar incidence rates among various ethnic groups living in the US. Among 53 patients with HIV-related PTCL collected from the records of investigators in Europe and the US and combined into a single analysis, 21 (42%) were Caucasian, 20 (40%) were Hispanic, 5 (10%) were African-American and 4 patients (8%) were of Asian descent. [6] However, until comprehensive and geographically diverse data bases are available, accurate inferences regarding disparities in ARTCL incidence between various ethnic or racial groups will remain-incomplete.

At time of medical diagnosis, 70-90% of patients with ARL have systemic 'B' symptoms consisting of fever, drenching night sweats and unintentional weight loss greater than 10% of ideal body weight. [5, 6, 21, 22] Like patients with AIDS-related BCLs, 75% of those with TCLs also present with stage III-IV disease. [5, 6]

Virtually any anatomic site may be involved by TCL. Rare cases of ARTCL involving the muscle, bone, kidneys, heart and adrenal glands have been reported. [5, 23] The majority of patients with ARTCL present with extranodal involvement. In one representative case series, 83% of all HIV-infected patients with TCLs had an extranodal component; only 17% were purely nodal. [13]

Reported sites of extranodal involvement include head and neck (23%), lungs (15%), gastrointestinal tract (14%), skin (9%) and CNS (9%). [13, 24] When compared to B-cell ARLs, ARTCLs have a higher likelihood of bone marrow (30-45% vs. 15%) and cutaneous (36% vs. 2%) involvement. [5] This is similar to the greater frequency of cutaneous and bone marrow involvement that occurs in non-HIV infected TCL patients, when compared to their B-cell lymphoma counterparts. [25-27]

Serum LDH levels are elevated in approximately 70% of patients with ARTCL. [6, 13] In the pre-HAART era, most of these patients were also more likely to have low CD4+ T-cell counts and elevated HIV viral loads. In a representative study of HIV-associated peripheral TCL, the median CD4+ count was 173 cells/mm^3 and the HIV viral load was 334,787 copies/mL. [6]

In another series, the median CD4+ count and HIV viral load at the time of lymphoma diagnosis was 130 cells/mm^3 (range, 15-1,578 cell/mm^3) and 279,185 copies/ml (range, undetectable to 600,000 copies/mm^3), respectively. [13] For patients who are receiving effective HAART and who have achieved immune reconstitution, a precipitous decline in CD4+ cell counts and B symptoms may be the initial harbingers of TCL. Opportunistic infections with *Candida*, *Mycobacterium* species and *Pneumocystis jiroveci* are frequently diagnosed in patients with ARTCL. Major clinical characteristics of ARTCL are listed in Table 5. [6]

The time interval between HIV diagnosis and diagnosis of ARTCL is not clearly defined. In a multicenter retrospective analysis of 39 ARTCL, the median time from HIV diagnosis to PTCL diagnosis was 4.5 years (range, 0-231 months). [6] Twelve (32%) of the patients had a diagnosis of AIDS and 10 (25%) were on HAART prior to their diagnosis of TCL. The impact of HAART on this latency interval is unknown.

Table 5. Clinical characteristics of AIDS-related T-cell lymphoma

Characteristic (n=cases with available data)	Number/median	Percentage/range
Age, years (n=51)	38	16-63
Sex (n=51)		
Male	42	82%
Female	9	18%
CD4+counts (n=38)		
< 200 cells/mm^3	27	71%
< 100 cells/mm^3	21	55%
< 50 cells/mm^3	11	29%
Performance status (n=49)		
ECOG 0-1	26	53%
ECOG $\geq$ 2	23	47%
LDH levels (n=37)		
Normal	12	32%
Elevated	25	68%
Clinical stage (n=51)		
Early stage (I - II)	13	25%
Advanced stage (III - IV)	38	75%
B symptoms (n=50)		
Absent	17	34%
Present	33	66%

Adapted from Castillo JJ, Beltran BE, et al. Prognostic factors in pateints with HIV-associated peripheral T-cell lymphoma: A multicenter study. *Am. J. Hematol.* 2011; 86:256.

Diagnosis of ARTCL requires expert examination of tissue including a detailed phenotypic assessment. Clonality should be assessed by polymerase chain reaction (PCR) for T-cell receptor gene rearrangements. [28] Staging evaluation should include computed tomographic scanning of the chest, abdomen and pelvis with or without positron emission tomography (PET) scan, and a marrow aspirate, biopsy and culture, including special stains for acid fast bacilli and fungus. Complete blood counts, chemistry tests and liver function tests and LDH, hepatitis serologies, CD4+ cell count and HIV viral load should also be collected. Other studies should be pursued as clinically indicated (e.g., retinal examination in patients with visual acuity changes, bronchoscopy for pulmonary infiltrates, etc.) in the context of advanced immunodeficiency. For those patients who are to be treated with an anthracycline, an echocardiogram to assess left ventricular function is routine. Unlike AIDS-related B-cell lymphomas, leptomeningeal and brain parenchymal involvement is uncommon in the setting of ARTCL. Consequently, in the absence of focal neurologic symptoms or signs, lumbar puncture and magnetic resonance imaging of the brain are not routinely pursued.

Diagnosis and management of patients with ARTCLs is complex, and the social difficulties that these patients may be experiencing can be extremely challenging. Care is best delivered with the support of a multidisciplinary team. The team should ideally include an Infectious Disease specialist, a Medical Social Worker or a Case Manager, and a Hematologist/Oncologist with special interest in both lymphomas and the care of PLWHA. Those patients requiring treatment should generally be referred to a cancer or tertiary care center with HIV/AIDS expertise.

PROGNOSIS

TCLs are not only rare but the various subtypes are heterogeneous with regards to clinical presentation and histopathology findings. Furthermore, these lymphoma subtypes have, with the exception of ALK-positive ALCL, generally been associated with a poor clinical outcome. [8] In a comprehensive literature review of multiple case reports and small case series, 72% of patients with ARTCL died; their median *o*verall *s*urvival (OS) time was only 6 months. [13] PTCL-U was associated with the longest median OS of 9 months, followed by ALCL at 6 months. With a median OS of 2.5 months and 1.5 months, respectively, the PCNSL and NK-TCL subtypes had the shortest median survival times. The cause of death was most frequently because of refractory or progressive lymphoma and/or infection. In contrast, in a multicenter retrospective analysis of ARTCL, the median OS was approximately 12 months, with no statistical survival difference among different ARTCL subtypes. [6] The reasons for disparity in survival between these studies is uncertain but may be related to HIV specific and tumor specific differences between the cohorts.

The median OS of patients with ARTCL appears to be shorter than those of their non-HIV-infected counterparts; wherein, the reported 5-year OS is 32%. [8] A small case series compared the survival of patients with HIV-associated BCL and HIV-associated TCL and found no statistical difference. [5] However, in that study, only 15% of the patients had received HAART and CD4+ cell counts were very low (<100 cells/mm^3) in both groups. Further studies are needed to clarify these observations in the HAART era.

Several prognostic factors have been described in ARLs, and they have been subdivided into HIV-related and lymphoma-related factors. Among the HIV-related factors, low CD4+ cell counts and the lack of effective HAART have been associated with diminished survival. [29, 30]

Additional adverse prognostic factors have also included presence of active opportunistic infections around the time of lymphoma diagnosis, age greater than 60 years old, and concurrent intravenous drug use. Among the lymphoma-related factors, the most widely used risk-stratification tool is the *I*nternational *P*rognostic *I*ndex (IPI) score. [30-32] The IPI score is routinely used to risk-stratify BCL, and in a prospective study was also validated as a prognostic tool in ARL. [33] The IPI score has been used less frequently in the context of TCL, but it too has been validated as a prognostic tool in this context. [30, 34]

Attempts have been made to define biologically distinct subgroups of TCL based upon clinical, biological and molecular prognostic factors. A *P*rognostic *I*ndex for P*T*CL-U (PIT) score based on age greater than 60 years, Eastern Co-operative Oncology Group (ECOG) performance status ≥ 2, elevated LDH and presence of bone marrow involvement have been validated in immune-competent patients. [35] Among 35 patients with ARTCL, 18 (51%) had a high PIT score (≥ 2 factors), while 17 (49%) patients had a low score (0-1 factors). [6]

It is uncertain whether lymphoma-related factors are stronger prognosticators than HIV related factors; it is likely that both play a role in predicting survival in ARLs. In the multicenter study of ARTCL patients, the univariate analysis showed that two HIV-related factors (CD4+ cell count and use of HAART) and three lymphoma-related factors (presence of B symptoms, IPI score and PIT score) were associated with OS. [7] Multivariate analysis showed that the use of HAART was independently associated with a better OS. while an ECOG performance status ≥ 2 was associated with a worse OS (Table 6).

Table 6. Univariate and Multivariate Survival Analysis of patients with AIDS-related T-cell lymphoma

Variable	Univariate analysis		Multivariate analysis	
	HR (95% CI)	P-value	HR (95% CI)	P-value
Male sex	1.1 (0.5–2.9)	NS		
CD4+ count <200 cells/mm^3	3.4 (1.4–8.1)	0.03		
Use of HAART	0.3 (0.1–0.9)	0.003	0.3 (0.1–0.8)	0.01
Presence of B symptoms	2.0 (0.9–4.2)	NS		
Performance status ECOG ≥ 2	3.1 (1.5–6.7)	0.001	3.4 (1.4–8.1)	0.007
>1 extranodal sites	1.2 (0.6–2.5)	NS		
Bone marrow involvement	0.5 (0.2–1.4)	NS		
Clinical stage 3–4	1.0 (0.4–2.2)	NS		
Elevated LDH levels	0.9 (0.3–2.5)	NS		
aaIPI score 2–3	2.5 (1.0–6.1)	0.025		
PIT score 2–4	3.9 (1.5–10.0)	0.004		

CI: confidence interval; ECOG: Eastern Cooperative Oncology Group; HAART: highly active. antiretroviral therapy; HR: hazard ratio; LDH: lactate dehydrogenase; aaIPI: age-adjusted. International Prognostic Index; PIT: Prognostic Index for PTCL, unspecified; NS: not significant.

Adapted from Castillo JJ, Beltran BE, et al. Prognostic factors in pateints with HIV-associated peripheral T-cell lymphoma: A multicenter study. *Am. J. Hematol.* 2011; 86:25.

The use of HAART and the enhanced immunological response that these combination antivirals induce has not only been associated with a decrease in the incidence but also an improvement in survival of patients with HIV-associated lymphomas. [36, 37] Nonetheless, concerns regarding drug interactions between HAART and chemotherapy are still being defined. [38]

TREATMENT

The treatment of ARTCLs involves overcoming several problems. These are aggressive lymphomas which typically present with advanced stage disease including bone marrow and extranodal involvement. Even with multiagent chemotherapy and state-of-the-art supportive care. response rates and complete remissions are suboptimal. In addition, the immunodeficiency of AIDS and the leukopenia that is commonly seen with HIV infection makes the use of immunosuppressive chemotherapy more problematic than in the non-HIV setting.

The treatment of patients with ARL, in general, presents the challenge of integrating therapy appropriate for the stage and histologic subset of lymphoma with the limitations imposed by HIV infection. Largely, the treatment approaches are similar to various subtypes of TCL with the exception of NK-TCL, where involved-field radiation, typically without chemotherapy, appears to be the key treatment modality. [13] In addition to antitumor therapy, essential components of an optimal non-Hodgkin lymphoma treatment strategy include the following: HAART; prophylaxis for opportunistic infections; and rapid recognition and treatment of intercurrent infections. [39]

The uncertainty of how chemotherapy drugs might interact with the various potential HAART options is also daunting. There are now 24 distinct drugs approved by the US Food and Drug Administration for treatment of HIV/AIDS. Classes of antiretroviral drugs include nucleoside reverse-transcriptase inhibitors (NRTIs), non-nucleoside reverse-transcriptase inhibitors (NNRTIs), HIV protease inhibitors, integrase strand-transfer inhibitors (INSTIs), fusion inhibitors, and entry inhibitors including chemokine-receptor antagonists. (Table 7) HAART typically consists of a combination of three active drugs which act on varied areas of the HIV lifecycle.

The most common choices for upfront therapy include a combination of two NRTIs with an NNRTI, a ritonavir-boosted protease inhibitor or an INSTI. Some NRTI-based or NNRTI-based regimens are associated with anemia, dyslipidemia, gastrointestinal symptoms, insulin resistance, neutropenia, nephrotoxicity, lactic acidosis, non-cirrhotic portal hypertension, pancreatitis, peripheral neuropathy and increased risk of thrombosis. In this context, Oncologists and HIV specialists need to be mindful of potential cancer drugs that rely on the CYP hepatic microsome pathways for degradation. [38]

Patients with widespread TCL may be treated with a combination of chemotherapeutic agents, including anthracycline-based regimens, which carry variable response rates and high rates of relapse. [40] Several case reports and case series have been reported results with the following regimens: CHOP (cyclophosphamide, doxorubicin, vincristine and prednisone); CDE (cyclophosphamide, doxorubicin and etoposide); PVB (cisplatin, vinblastine and bleomycin); ESHAP (etoposide, methylprednisolone, cisplatin and cytarabine); ABVD (doxorubicin, bleomycin, vinblastine and dacarbazine); CVP (cyclophosphamide, vincristine and prednisone); ICE (ifosfamide, carboplatin and etoposide) and ACVB (doxorubicin, cyclophosphamide, vindesine, bleomycin and prednisone). [6] The most common regimen employed for treatment of ARTCL is CHOP. [5, 6, 13] In a recent multicenter study of ARTCL, the OR rate to chemotherapy was about 65% with a 43% complete response (CR) and 21% partial response (PR). Progressive disease (PD) was seen in 36% of patients. [6]

Those patients who achieve a CR are more likely to have earlier stage disease, no bone marrow or CNS involvement, no prior AIDS-defining illness, and a good ECOG performance status. [6] Patients at risk for rare CNS involvement include those with bone marrow involvement or those with EBV identified in the primary tumor or in the cerebrospinal fluid. [41] Intrathecal chemotherapy is recommended for those patients at heightened risk for CNS involvement.

The introduction of HAART has led to a marked reduction in opportunistic infections, and also has contributed to prolonged survival for PLWHA. In the HAART era, the median OS for patients with AIDS-related lymphoma is now comparable to the outcome in the non-immunosuppressed population. [31, 37, 41-46] The use of HAART has made it easier for the use of standard dose and dose-intensive chemotherapy regimens to be given with reasonable safety to patients with AIDS-related lymphomas. 31, 37, 41-45]

Use of salvage second line chemotherapy, followed by autologous hematopoietic stem cell transplant in patients with resistant or relapsed ARCL has been anecdotally reported. [6, 47] As is true of the non-HIV infected population, further studies are needed to better define the timing and role of high-dose chemotherapy followed by stem cell transplant either as an upfront option or as a salvage after an incomplete response to initial treatment and at time of relapse.

The paucity of cases of ARTCL makes this a daunting task. No doubt, novel treatment approaches (e.g., pralatrexate, histone deacetylase inhibitors, proteasome inhibitors, and monoclonal antibodies, e.g., brentuximab vedotin) which are quickly being adopted in the non-HIV setting will find use in the context of ARTCL.

Table 7. Classification of HIV antiretroviral drugs

Drug (abbreviations)	Brand name
Nucleoside and nucleotide reverse transcriptase inhibitors (NRTIs)	
Abacavir (ABC)	Ziagen®
Didanosine (ddI)	Videx®, Videx® EC
Emtricitabine (FTC)	Emtriva®
Lamivudine (3TC)	Epivir®
Stavudine (d4T)	Zerit®
Tenofovir (TDF)	Viread®*
Zalcitabine (ddC)	Hivid®
Zidovudine (ZDV, AZT)	Retrovir®
Non-nucleoside reverse transcriptase inhibitors (NNRTIs)	
Delavirdine (DLV)	Rescriptor®
Efavirenz (EFV)	Sustiva®
Nevirapine (NVP)	Viramune®
Rilpivirine (RPV)	Edurant®
Protease inhibitors (PIs)	
Amprenavir (APV)	Agenerase®
Atazanavir (ATV)	Reyataz®
Darunavir (DRV)	Prezista®
Fosamprenavir (FPV)	Lexiva®
Indinavir (IDV)	Crixivan®
Lopinavir/ritonavir (LPV/r)	Kaletra®
Nelfinavir (NFV)	Viracept®
Ritonavir (RTV)	Norvir®
Saquinavir (SQV)	Fortovase®, Invirase®
Tipranavir (TPV)	Aptivus®
Fusion inhibitor	
Enfuvirtide (T-20)	Fuzeon®
Integrase inhibitor	
Raltegravir (RAL)	Isentress®
CCR5 antagonist	
Maraviroc (MVC)	Salzentry®
Fixed dose combinations	
Zidovudine + Lamivudine	Combivir®
Zidovudine + Lamivudine + Abacavir	Trizivir®
Lamivudine + Abacavir	Epzicom®
Emtricitabine + Tenofovir	Truvada®

Conclusion

In comparison to B-cell ARL, there is very limited published scientific literature on ARTCL. This group of lymphomas represents a diagnostic and therapeutic challenge for clinicians. The diversity of the various T-cell subtypes and the variety of viral pathogens that have been linked to their etiopathogenesis suggests dysfunction of immune system and viral oncogenes as common factors that may contribute to the heightened risk of TCL in PLWHA. To what extent HIV itself plays a role in pathogenesis of these lymphomas remains to be determined. Much work is needed to improve prognostic and therapeutic approaches of ARTCL.

Novel agents currently being investigated in the context of non-HIV associated TCL will have an important role in the treatment of ARTCL. These drugs will need to be studied carefully in the setting of HIV infection. Oncologists and HIV specialists will need to work together to manage patients with ARTCL and define the safety and efficacy of novel chemotherapy agents and how best to incorporate these newer drugs with our increasing large array of HAART options.

References

[1] 1993 Revised Classification System for HIV Infection and Expanded Surveillance Case Definition for AIDS Among Adolescents and Adults 1992; http://www.cdc.gov/mmwr/preview/mmwrhtml/00018871.htm. Accessed 05/10/2012.

[2] SEER Stat Fact Sheets: T-cell Non-Hodgkin Lymphoma. http://seer.cancer.gov/statfacts/html/tcellnhl.html. Accessed 05/10/2012, 2012.

[3] Patel P, Hanson DL, Sullivan PS, et al. Incidence of types of cancer among HIV-infected persons compared with the general population in the United States, 1992-2003. *Annals of internal medicine.* May 20 2008;148(10):728-736.

[4] Cote TR, Biggar RJ, Rosenberg PS, et al. Non-Hodgkin's lymphoma among people with AIDS: incidence, presentation and public health burden. AIDS/Cancer Study Group. *International journal of cancer. Journal international du cancer.* Nov 27 1997; 73(5):645-650.

[5] Arzoo KK, Bu X, Espina BM, Seneviratne L, Nathwani B, Levine AM. T-cell lymphoma in HIV-infected patients. *J Acquir Immune Defic Syndr.* Aug 15 2004; 36(5): 1020-1027.

[6] Castillo JJ, Beltran BE, Bibas M, et al. Prognostic factors in patients with HIV-associated peripheral T-cell lymphoma: a multicenter study. *American journal of hematology.* Mar 2011;86(3):256-261.

[7] Biggar RJ, Engels EA, Frisch M, Goedert JJ. Risk of T-cell lymphomas in persons with AIDS. *J Acquir Immune Defic Syndr.* Apr 1 2001;26(4):371-376.

[8] Vose J, Armitage J, Weisenburger D. International peripheral T-cell and natural killer/T-cell lymphoma study: pathology findings and clinical outcomes. *Journal of clinical oncology: official journal of the American Society of Clinical Oncology.* Sep 1 2008;26(25):4124-4130.

[9] Martin JN, Ganem DE, Osmond DH, Page-Shafer KA, Macrae D, Kedes DH. Sexual transmission and the natural history of human herpesvirus 8 infection. *The New England journal of medicine.* Apr 2 1998;338(14):948-954.
[10] Carbone A, Gloghini A. AIDS-related lymphomas: from pathogenesis to pathology. *British journal of haematology.* Sep 2005;130(5):662-670.
[11] Nakajima K, Martinez-Maza O, Hirano T, et al. Induction of IL-6 (B cell stimulatory factor-2/IFN-beta 2) production by HIV. *J Immunol.* Jan 15 1989;142(2):531-536.
[12] Carbone A, Gloghini A, Dotti G. EBV-associated lymphoproliferative disorders: classification and treatment. *The oncologist.* May 2008;13(5):577-585.
[13] Castillo JJ, Perez K, Milani C, Dezube BJ, Pantanowitz L. Peripheral T-cell lymphomas in HIV-infected individuals: a comprehensive review. *Journal of HIV Therapy.* 2009; 14(2):7.
[14] Du MQ, Bacon CM, Isaacson PG. Kaposi sarcoma-associated herpesvirus/human herpesvirus 8 and lymphoproliferative disorders. *Journal of clinical pathology.* Dec 2007; 60(12):1350-1357.
[15] van Tienen C, Schim van der Loeff M, Peterson I, et al. HTLV-1 and HIV-2 infection are associated with increased mortality in a rural West African community. *PloS one.* 2011; 6(12):e29026.
[16] Franceschi S, Lise M, Clifford GM, et al. Changing patterns of cancer incidence in the early- and late-HAART periods: the Swiss HIV Cohort Study. *British journal of cancer.* Jul 27 2010;103(3):416-422.
[17] Polesel J, Clifford GM, Rickenbach M, et al. Non-Hodgkin lymphoma incidence in the Swiss HIV Cohort Study before and after highly active antiretroviral therapy. *AIDS.* Jan 11 2008;22(2):301-306.
[18] Swerdlow SH, Campo E, Harris NL, et al. *World Health Organization Classification of Tumours of Haematopoietic and Lymphoid Tissues.* Vol 2. Lyon: IARC Press; 2008.
[19] Castillo J, Pantanowitz L, Dezube BJ. HIV-associated plasmablastic lymphoma: lessons learned from 112 published cases. *American journal of hematology.* Oct 2008; 83(10): 804-809.
[20] Luther VP, Wilkin AM. HIV infection in older adults. *Clinics in geriatric medicine.* Aug 2007;23(3):567-583, vii.
[21] Levine AM. Acquired immunodeficiency syndrome-related lymphoma. *Blood.* Jul 1 1992; 80(1): 8-20.
[22] Levine AM, Sullivan-Halley J, Pike MC, et al. Human immunodeficiency virus-related lymphoma. Prognostic factors predictive of survival. *Cancer.* Dec 1 1991;68(11):2466-2472.
[23] Pantanowitz L, Castillo J, Freeman JK, Dezube BJ. Images in HIV/AIDS. Fatal HIV-associated anaplastic large-cell lymphoma. *The AIDS reader.* Jan 2009; 19(1): 19-21.
[24] Perez K, Castillo J, Dezube BJ, Pantanowitz L. Human Immunodeficiency Virus-associated anaplastic large cell lymphoma. *Leukemia and lymphoma.* Mar 2010;51(3): 430-438.
[25] Gisselbrecht C, Gaulard P, Lepage E, et al. Prognostic significance of T-cell phenotype in aggressive non-Hodgkin's lymphomas. Groupe d'Etudes des Lymphomes de l'Adulte (GELA). *Blood.* Jul 1 1998;92(1):76-82.

[26] Lippman SM, Miller TP, Spier CM, Slymen DJ, Grogan TM. The prognostic significance of the immunotype in diffuse large-cell lymphoma: a comparative study of the T-cell and B-cell phenotype. *Blood.* Aug 1988;72(2):436-441.

[27] Lopez-Guillermo A, Cid J, Salar A, et al. Peripheral T-cell lymphomas: initial features, natural history, and prognostic factors in a series of 174 patients diagnosed according to the R.E.A.L. Classification. *Annals of oncology: official journal of the European Society for Medical Oncology / ESMO.* Aug 1998;9(8):849-855.

[28] Dearden CE, Johnson R, Pettengell R, et al. Guidelines for the management of mature T-cell and NK-cell neoplasms (excluding cutaneous T-cell lymphoma). *British journal of haematology.* May 2011;153(4):451-485.

[29] Simcock M, Blasko M, Karrer U, et al. Treatment and prognosis of AIDS-related lymphoma in the era of highly active antiretroviral therapy: findings from the Swiss HIV Cohort Study. *Antiviral therapy.* 2007;12(6):931-939.

[30] Miralles P, Berenguer J, Ribera JM, et al. Prognosis of AIDS-related systemic non-Hodgkin lymphoma treated with chemotherapy and highly active antiretroviral therapy depends exclusively on tumor-related factors. *J Acquir Immune Defic Syndr.* Feb 1 2007;44(2):167-173.

[31] Mounier N, Spina M, Gabarre J, et al. AIDS-related non-Hodgkin lymphoma: final analysis of 485 patients treated with risk-adapted intensive chemotherapy. *Blood.* May 15 2006;107(10):3832-3840.

[32] Tanaka PY, Pracchia LF, Bellesso M, Chamone DA, Calore EE, Pereira J. A prognostic score for AIDS-related diffuse large B-cell lymphoma in Brazil. *Annals of hematology.* Jun 4 2009.

[33] A predictive model for aggressive non-Hodgkin's lymphoma. The International Non-Hodgkin's Lymphoma Prognostic Factors Project. *The New England journal of medicine.* Sep 30 1993;329(14):987-994.

[34] Ansell SM, Habermann TM, Kurtin PJ, et al. Predictive capacity of the International Prognostic Factor Index in patients with peripheral T-cell lymphoma. *Journal of clinical oncology : official journal of the American Society of Clinical Oncology.* Jun 1997; 15(6):2296-2301.

[35] Gallamini A, Stelitano C, Calvi R, et al. Peripheral T-cell lymphoma unspecified (PTCL-U): a new prognostic model from a retrospective multicentric clinical study. *Blood.* Apr 1 2004;103(7):2474-2479.

[36] Ribera JM, Navarro JT. Human immunodeficiency virus-related non-Hodgkin's lymphoma. *Haematologica.* Aug 2008;93(8):1129-1132.

[37] Hoffmann C, Wolf E, Fatkenheuer G, et al. Response to highly active antiretroviral therapy strongly predicts outcome in patients with AIDS-related lymphoma. *AIDS.* Jul 4 2003; 17(10):1521-1529.

[38] Rudek MA, Flexner C, Ambinder RF. Use of antineoplastic agents in patients with cancer who have HIV/AIDS. *The lancet oncology.* Sep 2011;12(9):905-912.

[39] Vishnu P, Aboulafia DM. AIDS-Related Non-Hodgkin's Lymphoma in the Era of Highly Active Antiretroviral Therapy. *Advances in hematology.* 2012;2012:485943.

[40] Rizvi MA, Evens AM, Tallman MS, Nelson BP, Rosen ST. T-cell non-Hodgkin lymphoma. *Blood.* Feb 15 2006;107(4):1255-1264.

[41] Cingolani A, Gastaldi R, Fassone L, et al. Epstein-Barr virus infection is predictive of CNS involvement in systemic AIDS-related non-Hodgkin's lymphomas. *Journal of*

clinical oncology: official journal of the American Society of Clinical Oncology. Oct 1 2000;18(19):3325-3330.

[42] Palella FJ, Jr., Delaney KM, Moorman AC, et al. Declining morbidity and mortality among patients with advanced human immunodeficiency virus infection. HIV Outpatient Study Investigators. *The New England journal of medicine.* Mar 26 1998; 338(13): 853-860.

[43] Tam HK, Zhang ZF, Jacobson LP, et al. Effect of highly active antiretroviral therapy on survival among HIV-infected men with Kaposi sarcoma or non-Hodgkin lymphoma. *International journal of cancer. Journal international du cancer.* Apr 20 2002;98(6): 916-922.

[44] Vaccher E, Spina M, Talamini R, et al. Improvement of systemic human immunodeficiency virus-related non-Hodgkin lymphoma outcome in the era of highly active antiretroviral therapy. *Clinical infectious diseases : an official publication of the Infectious Diseases Society of America.* Dec 1 2003;37(11):1556-1564.

[45] Weiss R, Mitrou P, Arasteh K, et al. Acquired immunodeficiency syndrome-related lymphoma: simultaneous treatment with combined cyclophosphamide, doxorubicin, vincristine, and prednisone chemotherapy and highly active antiretroviral therapy is safe and improves survival--results of the German Multicenter Trial. *Cancer.* Apr 1 2006; 106(7):1560-1568.

[46] Wolf T, Brodt HR, Fichtlscherer S, et al. Changing incidence and prognostic factors of survival in AIDS-related non-Hodgkin's lymphoma in the era of highly active antiretroviral therapy (HAART). *Leukemia and lymphoma.* Feb 2005;46(2):207-215.

[47] Balsalobre P, Diez-Martin JL, Re A, et al. Autologous stem-cell transplantation in patients with HIV-related lymphoma. *Journal of clinical oncology : official journal of the American Society of Clinical Oncology.* May 1 2009;27(13):2192-2198.

In: Hodgkin's and T-Cell Lymphoma
Editors: Warren K. Harvey and Randall M. Jacobs
ISBN 978-1-62257-478-0

Chapter 6

CRITICAL MASS HYPOTHESIS OF T-CELL RESPONSES AND ITS APPLICATION FOR THE TREATMENT OF T-CELL LYMPHOMA

***Christopher Bricogne*[1], *Roberta Laranga*[1], *Antonella Padella*[1], *Ines Dufait*[1,2], *Therese Liechtenstein*[1], *Karine Breckpot*[2], *Grazyna Kochan*[3] and *David Escors*[1*]**

[1]Division of Infection and Immunity, Rayne Institute, University College London, London. UK
[2]Laboratory of Molecular and Cellular Therapy, Department of Physiology-Immunology, Medical School of the Vrije Universiteit Brussel, Jette, Belgium
[3]Structural Genomics Consortium Oxford, University of Oxford, Headington, Oxford, UK

ABSTRACT

Adaptive immune responses against intracellular pathogens and cancer must find a balance between the effective elimination of target cells on one hand, and collateral damage to healthy tissues on the other. Precise and subtle timing of effector activity is vital to achieving this balance. Ligand-induced TCR down-modulation, whereby T cell receptors (TCR) are removed from the surface shortly after engagement with peptide-MHC (p-MHC), has been extensively studied over the past 20 years; however this critical process is still poorly understood, and both the underlying mechanism and its physiological significance remain unclear. Most experimental evidence supports that TCR down-modulation attenuates T cell activation by removing TCRs from the T cell surface, thereby limiting TCR signal transduction and preventing cell hyper-activation and hazardous inflammation. Here, we put forward a complementary hypothesis. TCRs are down-modulated after antigen presentation and remain so during the exponential

* Corresponding author: David Escors. E-mail: d.escors@ucl.ac.uk

phase of effector T cell expansion. Then, TCRs are re-expressed as T cell numbers reach their peak. In this way the initiation of cytotoxic responses can be synchronised with the time at which a "critical mass" of effector T cells has accumulated. Therefore, TCR down-modulation co-ordinates cytotoxic function with effector capacity, reducing the likelihood of untimely cytotoxic activity which could give rise to autoimmune disease. We discuss the therapeutic implications of targeting TCR down-modulation and modifying the kinetics of T cell responses, with an emphasis on their application for immunotherapy of T cell lymphoma.

INTRODUCTION

The expansion of antigen-specific cytotoxic CD8 T cells plays a critical role in achieving long-lasting immunity against infectious diseases and cancer (Boon and van der Bruggen, 1996; Breckpot et al, 2003; Breckpot and Escors, 2009; Firat et al, 1999; He et al, 2005; Morgan et al, 2006; Van den Eynde and van der Bruggen, 1997). Cytotoxic T cells are activated after encountering their specific cognate antigen during antigen presentation. This involves recognition of antigenic peptides associated with major histocompatibility complexes (p-MHC) on the surface of antigen presenting cells (APCs). T cells bind to these p-MHC complexes *via* their antigen-specific TCR, triggering their activation, clonal expansion and acquisition of effector functions.

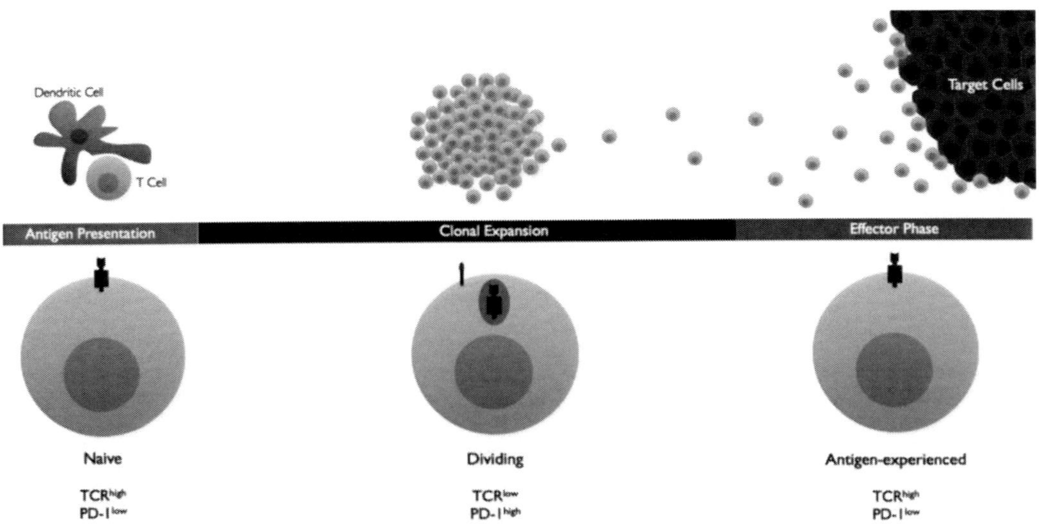

Figure 1. The three phases of the anti-tumour T cell response. The scheme depicts the three phases of T cell responses in tumour immunotherapy, starting on the left with antigen presentation. DCs present antigen to T cells, which express high levels of surface TCR and low levels of PD-1. In the centre, activated T cells expand exponentially. During this phase, TCRs are removed from the surface while PD-1 is expressed at high levels. This process takes about one week. In the effector phase (right), a critical mass of effector T cells has been reached. These T cells re-express the antigen-specific TCR. As a consequence of their activation by antigen presentation, they still express a significant amount of PD-1, although it is progressively down-modulated. These T cells recognise their cellular targets in the form of tumour-associated antigens presented on the surface of cancer cells. The p-MHC recognition triggers their cytotoxic activities.

However, the actions of cytotoxic T cells cause significant "collateral damage" to bystander tissues by potentiating inflammation. This increases the chances of inducing autoimmune pathology if inadequately controlled. Thus, T cell responses must be tightly regulated at different levels. One of these key checkpoints in T cell activation is right at its origin during antigen presentation. APCs such as dendritic cells (DCs) process and expose antigenic peptides to potential effector T cells (Arce et al, 2011; Breckpot and Escors, 2009; Goold et al., 2011). Activated T cells undergo a rapid exponential clonal expansion before entering the effector phase when they eliminate the target cells (Figure 1).

1. The Three-Signal Model of T Cell Activation. Concept of Co-Stimulation

The interaction between the TCR and its cognate p-MHC alone is not sufficient for T cell activation, and must be accompanied by a number of auxiliary co-stimulatory signals. A wide range of ligand-receptor and cytokine-receptor interactions provides these signals that influence the magnitude and type of T cell responses. A "three-signal" model of T cell activation is widely accepted by immunologists. This model involves pMHC-TCR binding as delivering signal 1, and co-stimulatory (either "positive" or "negative") ligand-receptor interactions as signal 2.

The integration of stimulatory and inhibitory interactions (signal 2) dictates the magnitude of the T cell response (Nurieva et al, 2006). For example, CD28 binding on T cells to CD80/CD86 on DCs is potently stimulatory, while inhibitory signals are delivered by PD-1 binding to PD-L1.

In addition, a third signal polarises T cell differentiation into distinct T cell types, such as cytotoxic CD8 T cells, CD4 T helper (Th) 1, Th2, Th17 or T regulatory cells. This signal is generally provided in the form of secreted cytokines/chemokines, and it is sometimes referred as "cytokine priming" (Breckpot and Escors, 2009; Curtsinger et al., 2003; Curtsinger et al., 1999; Kalinski et al., 1999; Ramanathan et al., 2011; Ramanathan et al., 2010).

2. PD-L1/PD-1 Co-Stimulation in the Immunological Synapse and Ligand-Induced TCR Down-Modulation

"Negative co-stimulation" between the APC and T cells takes place regularly during antigen presentation. This is difficult to reconcile with the classical role of co-stimulation for T cell licensing and activation. One of such interactions occurs between PD-L1 in the APC surface with its receptor PD-1 on T cells, which suppresses TCR signal transduction and T cell activation (Freeman et al., 2000; Latchman et al., 2001). This is a strong T cell inhibitory interaction, and PD-L1/PD-1 interactions strongly interfere with anti-tumour immune responses in the tumour microenvironment and seem to participate in T cell exhaustion (Barber et al, 2006; Zhang et al., 2009). On the other hand, this interaction plays a key role in maintaining peripheral tolerance (Francisco et al., 2010; Latchman et al., 2004; Wang et al., 2008).

Table 1. Interference with PD-L1/PD-1 engagement results in autoimmune disorders

	IMMUNOPATHOLOGY	CHARACTER	SPECIES	REFERENCES
PD-1 -/-	Lupus-like autoimmune disease	Spontaneous	Mouse	Nishimura et al. Immunity, 1999
	Cardiomyopathy	Spontaneous	Mouse	Nishimura el al. Science, 2001
	Type 1 diabetes	Predisposition	Mouse	Ansari et al. J. Exp. Med., 2003
PD-1 blockade	Type I diabetes	Spontaneous	Mouse	Ansari et al. J. Exp. Med., 2003
	Graft vs host disease	Worsened	Mouse	Blazar et al. J. Immunol., 2003
	Experimental Autoimmune Encephalomyelitis	Worsened	Mouse	Salama et al. J. Exp. Med., 2003
PD-1 polymorphisms	Multiple sclerosis	Susceptibility	Human	Kroner et al, Ann Neurol, 2005
	Type I diabetes	Susceptibility	Human	Nielse et al, Tissue Antigens, 2003
	Systemic Lupus Erythematosus	Susceptibility	Human	Prokunina et al, Nat Genetics, 2002; Johansson et al, Arthritis Rheum, 2005; Wang et al, J Clin Immunol, 2006
	Lupus Nephritis	Susceptibility	Human	Prokunina et al, Arthritis Rheum, 2004
	Rheumatoid Arthritis	Susceptibility	Human	Kong et al, Arthritis Rheum, 2005; Prokunina et al, Arthritis Rheum, 2004; Lin et al, Arthritis Rheum, 2004
	Ankylosing Spondylitis	Susceptibility	Human	Lee et al, Arthritis Res Ther, 2006
Cbl-b -/-	Type I diabetes	Susceptibility	Rat	Yokoi et al, Nat Genetics, 2002
	Multisystem autoimmune disease	Spontaneous	Mouse	Myung-Shin et al, Immunity, 2004; Bachmaier et al, Nature, 2000
	Tumour rejection	Spontaneous	Mouse	Loeser et al, J. Exp. Med., 2007; Chiang et al, J Clin Invest, 2007
	Experimental Autoimmune Encephalomyelitis	Susceptibility	Mouse	Chiang et al, Nature, 2000

Consequently, an increased susceptibility to autoimmune disorders has been observed in virtually all KO mouse models targeting any component of the PD-L1/PD-1 signalling pathway (Table 1) (Bachmaier et al., 2000; Chiang et al., 2000; Francisco et al., 2010;

Latchman et al., 2004; Nishimura et al., 2001; Okazaki et al, 2003; Sharpe et al, 2007; Wang et al., 2005).

PD-1 engagement triggers the recruitment of SHP phosphatases to its cytoplasmic “switch domain" (inhibitory tyrosine switch motif, or ITSM), resulting in the de-phosphorylation of key signalling molecules of the TCR signal-transduction machinery (Chemnitz et al., 2004; Sheppard et al., 2004). In addition to this, it was demonstrated that PD-1 engagement in T cells up-regulated several transcription factors including BATF, an ATF-like transcription factor with broad T cell inhibitory activities (Quigley et al., 2010). This result shows that PD-1 inhibitory activities must act at additional levels other than the recruitment of SHP phosphatases.

PD-L1/PD-1 engagement also takes place during activation of naïve T cells after antigen presentation, and it is thought to be a mechanism that regulates the extent of T cell activation. Surprisingly, we have recently observed that PD-L1/PD-1 binding between antigen-presenting DCs and T cells enhances ligand-induced TCR down-modulation in the immunological synapse. Ligand-induced TCR down-modulation is the process by which TCRs are removed from the cell surface shortly after engagement with p-MHC complexes on APCs.

Two models have been proposed based on the assumption that TCR/CD28 stimulation is a sufficient trigger for TCR down-modulation. In the “serial triggering model”, a single p-MHC complex can serially associate and trigger a very high number of TCRs in the immunological synapse (Valitutti et al., 1995).

On the other hand, the “TCR co-modulation model” proposes that engaged, and subsequently endocytosed, TCRs mediate signal transduction that triggers down-modulation of non-engaged TCRs as well (San Jose et al., 2000).

Interestingly, silencing of PD-L1 on antigen-presenting DCs significantly reduced the extent of ligand-induced TCR down-modulation, suggesting that at least one extrinsic signal is implicated in TCR down-modulation (Escors et al., 2011; Karwacz et al., 2012; Karwacz et al., 2011).

Although TCR down-modulation has been extensively studied over the last 20 years, its molecular mechanism and physiological relevance are still under debate. While some experimental evidence suggests that TCR down-modulation is required for T cell activation (Hansen et al., 2011; Valitutti et al., 1995), other studies show that it terminates TCR signal transduction to prevent hyper-activation (Baniyash, 2004; Boding et al., 2009; Bonefeld et al., 2008; Karwacz et al., 2011; Liu et al., 2000; Naramura et al., 2002).

3. Physiological Role of TCR Down-Modulation. The Critical Mass of Effector T Cells

There is increasing evidence that PD-L1/PD-1 co-stimulation during antigen presentation represents an early control of T cell activities, as it has an overall inhibitory effect on T cell activation (Francisco et al., 2010; Freeman et al., 2000). Interference with any step of PD-L1/PD-1 co-stimulation or TCR down-modulation increases the susceptibility to autoimmune disorders (Andre et al., 1997; Bachmaier et al., 2000; Karwacz et al., 2011; Latchman et al., 2004; Naramura et al., 2002; Nishimura et al., 2001) (Table 1).

Interestingly, ligand-induced TCR down-modulation reaches its maximum level between day three to five after antigen presentation (Karwacz et al., 2011), which coincides with the exponential phase of clonal expansion of effector T cells (Homann et al., 2001). After that, TCR surface levels recover just as T cell expansion has reached its peak, "arming" the T cells and enabling them to exert their cytotoxic activities (Figure 1). Thus, ligand-induced TCR down-modulation removes surface TCRs from the expanding population of effector T cells. Consequently, interference with PD-L1/PD-1 engagement between APCs and T cells inhibits TCR down-modulation. This lack of PD-L1/PD-1 binding during antigen presentation results in hyperactive effector T cells which exert their cytotoxic activities earlier compared to antigen presentation in the presence of physiological PD-L1 levels (Figure 2).

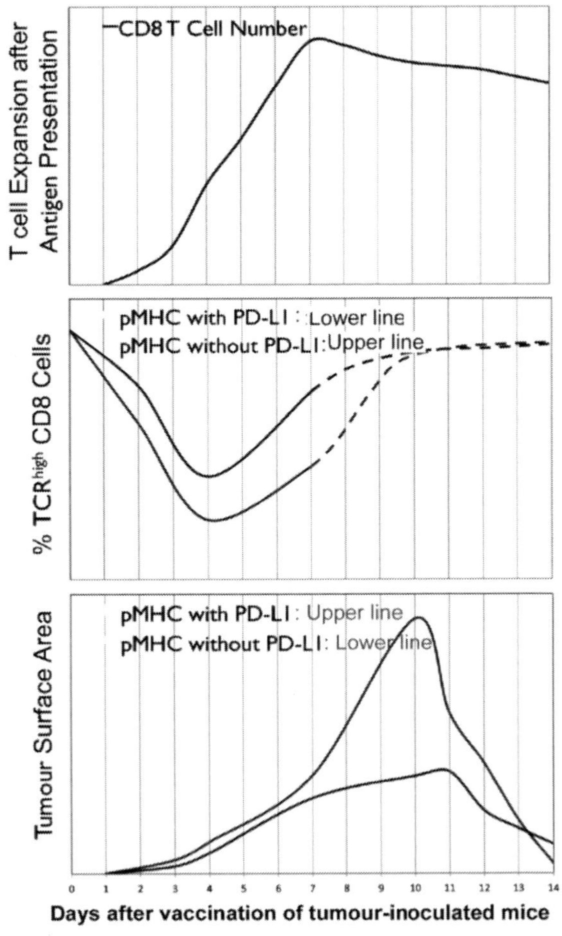

Figure 2. Separation of the antigen presentation phase from the effector phase by TCR down-modulation during an anti-lymphoma immune response. The expansion of antigen-specific CD8 T cells as a function of days after vaccination is plotted in the top graph. In the centre, TCR surface levels in expanding effector CD8 T cells are represented following the same timing as in the top graph. In the bottom graph, anti-tumour cytotoxic responses are monitored following the tumour surface area in tumour-inoculated mice (Karwacz et al., 2011). These mice were vaccinated with either wild-type or PD-L1-silenced DCs expressing the surrogate tumour antigen OVA. Mice were subcutaneously injected with a T cell lymphoma line expressing OVA (EG7 cells).

This suggests that removal of TCRs from expanding effector T cells circumvents their cytotoxicity until TCR surface expression is recovered. Work in other experimental systems supports this view, as effector T cells exhibit high cytotoxic activities only after recovering surface expression of their TCRs (Mannon et al., 1998).

This is quite an important observation, because TCR down-modulation would separate the antigen presentation phase from the effector phase. There are two stages in the life cycle of T cells where pMHC:TCR interactions occur: when T cells are activated by antigen-presenting DC, and when clonally expanded effector T cells encounter pMHC on target cells. While T cells regard pMHC as an activation signal during antigen presentation, effector T cells identify pMHC-bearing cells as the trigger for cytotoxic killing. A first consequence of TCR down-modulation is possibly the protection of antigen presenting DCs from attack. Secondly, any reduction in the number of dividing T cells at an early stage would decrease the eventual size of the expanded population.

Thus, another possible consequence of TCR down-modulation is that the effector phase is deferred, which would prevent the premature cytotoxic engagement of expanding T cells.

Finally, in order to minimise pathogen or malignant cell adaptation and resistance to an immune attack, a rapid, simultaneous and thorough "blitz" by all available cytotoxic T cells could be advantageous. A slow trickle of effector T cells would favour escape of tumour cells by providing time for selection of resistant malignant cells. Synchronisation of the peak in T cell numbers and of the onset of T cell functionality maximises the size and decreases the duration of the overall response.

Thus, PD-L1/PD-1 co-stimulation during T cell activation after antigen recognition might ensure that the timing of TCR down-modulation is in synchrony with the peak of effector T cell numbers. In the context of anti-tumour immunity, this is also the time at which tumour expansion ceases and regression begins to occur (Figure 2). This may explain why interference with PD-L1/PD-1 co-stimulation, thereby inhibiting TCR down-modulation, significantly accelerates anti-tumour activities and regression.

4. PD-L1/PD-1 Interference for Immunotherapy of T Cell Lymphoma

PD-L1/PD-1 interference or blockade *in vitro* is a promising approach for the treatment of viral chronic infections and tumour immunotherapy. However, interference with this interaction results in significant therapeutic improvement when combined with other immunotherapeutic strategies, radiotherapy and chemotherapy (Karwacz et al., 2012; Karwacz et al., 2011; Mangsbo et al., 2010; Stagg et al., 2011; Vezys et al., 2011).

PD-L1/PD-1 interaction plays a key immunosuppressive role in several types of T and B cell lymphomas, and PD-L1/PD-1 interference/blockade is currently being applied as an immunotherapeutic approach (Andorsky et al., 2011; Elpek et al., 2007; Green et al., 2010; Kozako et al., 2011; Kozako et al., 2009; Marzec et al., 2008; Samimi et al., 2010; Wilcox et al., 2009). This is particularly important since lymphoma cells up-regulate PD-L1 expression, which in turn inhibits the anti-tumour activities of infiltrating effector T cells (Andorsky et al., 2011; Samimi et al., 2010; Wilcox et al., 2009). In our recent publication (Escors et al., 2011; Karwacz et al., 2012; Karwacz et al., 2011), we tested whether silencing of PD-L1 in

DCs would improve immunotherapy for an aggressive MHC II negative T cell lymphoma model in mice. Our results demonstrated that interference with PD-L1/PD-1 interaction during antigen presentation inhibited TCR down-modulation. This was achieved by preventing the up-regulation of E3-ubiquitin ligases in activated CD8 T cells, which stops TCR signal transduction and induces TCR endocytosis. Interference with PD-L1 co-stimulation resulted in hyperactive TCR^{high} pro-inflammatory CD8 T cells, which accelerated the immune attack against an aggressive lymphoma model in mice. Surprisingly, the overall survival in mice vaccinated with PD-L1-silenced DCs did not significantly increase when compared with mice vaccinated with non-silenced DC vaccines. This result was surprising and unexpected, and suggested that even if the immune attack started earlier, it might not necessarily translate in more effective tumour eradication. It could well be that a sufficiently large T cell critical mass was not reached, and the overall T cell attack was insufficient to completely eliminate tumour cells. Thus, it might be possible that PD-L1/PD-1 interaction is after all required for an efficient anti-tumour immune response, even if an inhibitory receptor is strongly expressed in effector T cells. It is also well known that tumour cells can then up-regulate PD-L1, which could also switch off these anti-tumour T cells, adding an additional barrier for the efficacy of immunotherapy.

There are two possible solutions to overcome this problem while taking advantage of the T cell hyperactivity achieved by PD-L1/PD-1 blocking/interference. The first one is systemic administration of blocking antibodies, which would reach both tumour cells and APCs in the lymph node. These approaches have shown increased T cell infiltration in tumours and stronger association to APCs in tumour draining lymph nodes (Fife et al., 2009). The second approach is to increase the cytotoxic capacities of TCR^{high} CD8 T cells. This can be achieved by simultaneous inhibition of PD-L1 expression in DCs with expression of modulators of MAPK pathways that enhance antigen presentation. Thus, we showed that PD-L1 silencing in DCs combined with expression of a constitutive p38 activator (Escors et al., 2008), or a dominant negative MEK1 mutant, which inhibits ERK phosphorylation (Arce et al., 2011) resulted in accelerated anti-tumour immune responses with a significant increase in survival (Karwacz et al., 2011).

There are a number of clinical trials particularly for the treatment of melanoma and lung cancer, in which PD-L1/PD-1 blocking with antibodies increases survival in human patients. However, it has to be mentioned that these patients simultaneously receive chemotherapy/radiotherapy, treatments that also enhance immune responses (Apetoh et al., 2007; Arce et al., 2011; Finke et al., 2008; Ghiringhelli et al., 2009; Pilon-Thomas et al., 2010; Sakuishi et al., 2010; Xin et al., 2009; Zitvogel et al., 2008). It would be interesting to track and quantify T cell numbers and cytotoxic responses in patients receiving PD-L1/PD-1 blocking antibodies. It might be possible that the timing of administration could be critical for the enhancement of T cell activation without interference with T cell expansion.

CONCLUSION

In the critical mass hypothesis of T cell immunity, TCR down-modulation after antigen presentation synchronises the activity and expansion of effector T cells to maximise the killing potential of that expanded population. By transiently down-regulating TCR numbers on the cell surface, the onset of cytotoxic capacity of the T cells can be coordinated with the time at which a "critical mass" of effector T cells has been reached. We propose that this process is controlled through PD-L1/PD-1 engagement in the immunological synapse. PD-1 expression, ligation by PD-L1 and triggering of TCR down-regulation ensure (1) that the antigen-presenting DCs are not prematurely eliminated, (2) that newly activated, proliferating T cells are not limited in final effector population size due to untimely recruitment and (3) that malignant cells or intracellular pathogens are subjected to a "blitz" attack, being unable to adapt and evade the immune system.

Extensive research has been directed towards understanding the underlying regulatory processes that control the magnitude and character of T cell responses, so that targeted therapies can be designed to halt autoimmune disease or enhance immunity to cancer. The most fundamental regulatory checkpoint in the T cell response is at its origin, antigen presentation, when APCs activate T cells. The binding of pMHC:TCR triggers intracellular signalling cascades that result in T cell activation and proliferation. Auxiliary signals are also relayed via co-stimulatory ligands and cytokines that modulate TCR signalling. We propose that the role of PD-L1 extends beyond inhibiting intracellular signalling pathways through dephosphorylation. Through transiently down-regulating TCR numbers on the cell surface, the empowerment of effector T cells with their cytotoxic capacity can be synchronised with the time at which a critical mass of these cells has been produced. Our proposal may explain the physiological significance of ligand-induced TCR down-modulation, PD-L1 signalling and the importance of timing between activation, expansion and cytotoxic activities for an effective anti-tumour immune response.

References

Andorsky DJ, Yamada RE, Said J, Pinkus GS, Betting DJ, Timmerman JM (2011) Programmed death ligand 1 is expressed by non-hodgkin lymphomas and inhibits the activity of tumor associated T cells. *Clin. Cancer Res.* 17: 4232-4244.

Andre P, Boretto J, Hueber AO, Regnier-Vigouroux A, Gorvel JP, Ferrier P, Chavrier P (1997) A dominant-negative mutant of the Rab5 GTPase enhances T cell signaling by interfering with TCR down-modulation in transgenic mice. *Journal of immunology* 159: 5253-5263.

Apetoh L, Ghiringhelli F, Tesniere A, Obeid M, Ortiz C, Criollo A, Mignot G, Maiuri MC, Ullrich E, Saulnier P, Yang H, Amigorena S, Ryffel B, Barrat FJ, Saftig P, Levi F, Lidereau R, Nogues C, Mira JP, Chompret A, Joulin V, Clavel-Chapelon F, Bourhis J, Andre F, Delaloge S, Tursz T, Kroemer G, Zitvogel L (2007) Toll-like receptor 4-dependent contribution of the immune system to anticancer chemotherapy and radiotherapy. *Nat. Med.* 13: 1050-1059.

Arce F, Breckpot K, Stephenson H, Karwacz K, Ehrenstein MR, Collins M, Escors D (2011) Selective ERK activation differentiates mouse and human tolerogenic dendritic cells, expands antigen-specific regulatory T cells, and suppresses experimental inflammatory arthritis. *Arthritis and rheumatism* 63: 84-95.

Bachmaier K, Krawczyk C, Kozieradzki I, Kong YY, Sasaki T, Oliveira-dos-Santos A, Mariathasan S, Bouchard D, Wakeham A, Itie A, Le J, Ohashi PS, Sarosi I, Nishina H,

Lipkowitz S, Penninger JM (2000) Negative regulation of lymphocyte activation and autoimmunity by the molecular adaptor Cbl-b. *Nature* 403: 211-216.

Baniyash M (2004) TCR zeta-chain downregulation: curtailing an excessive inflammatory immune response. *Nature reviews Immunology* 4: 675-687.

Barber DL, Wherry EJ, Masopust D, Zhu B, Allison JP, Sharpe AH, Freeman GJ, Ahmed R (2006) Restoring function in exhausted CD8 T cells during chronic viral infection. *Nature* 439: 682-687.

Boding L, Bonefeld CM, Nielsen BL, Lauritsen JP, von Essen MR, Hansen AK, Larsen JM, Nielsen MM, Odum N, Geisler C (2009) TCR down-regulation controls T cell homeostasis. *Journal of immunology* 183: 4994-5005.

Bonefeld CM, Haks M, Nielsen B, von Essen M, Boding L, Hansen AK, Larsen JM, Odum N, Krimpenfort P, Kruisbeek A, Christensen JP, Thomsen AR, Geisler C (2008) TCR down-regulation controls virus-specific CD8+ T cell responses. *Journal of immunology* 181: 7786-7799.

Boon T, van der Bruggen P (1996) Human tumor antigens recognized by T lymphocytes. *J. Exp. Med.* 183: 725-729.

Breckpot K, Dullaers M, Bonehill A, van Meirvenne S, Heirman C, de Greef C, van der Bruggen P, Thielemans K (2003) Lentivirally transduced dendritic cells as a tool for cancer immunotherapy. *J. Gene Med.* 5: 654-667.

Breckpot K, Escors D (2009) Dendritic Cells for Active Anti-cancer Immunotherapy: Targeting Activation Pathways Through Genetic Modification. *Endocrine, metabolic and immune disorders drug targets* 9: 328-343.

Chemnitz JM, Parry RV, Nichols KE, June CH, Riley JL (2004) SHP-1 and SHP-2 associate with immunoreceptor tyrosine-based switch motif of programmed death 1 upon primary human T cell stimulation, but only receptor ligation prevents T cell activation. *J. Immunol.* 173: 945-954.

Chiang YJ, Kole HK, Brown K, Naramura M, Fukuhara S, Hu RJ, Jang IK, Gutkind JS, Shevach E, Gu H (2000) Cbl-b regulates the CD28 dependence of T-cell activation. *Nature* 403: 216-220.

Curtsinger JM, Lins DC, Mescher MF (2003) Signal 3 determines tolerance versus full activation of naive CD8 T cells: dissociating proliferation and development of effector function. *The Journal of experimental medicine* 197: 1141-1151.

Curtsinger JM, Schmidt CS, Mondino A, Lins DC, Kedl RM, Jenkins MK, Mescher MF (1999) Inflammatory cytokines provide a third signal for activation of naive CD4+ and CD8+ T cells. *Journal of immunology* 162: 3256-3262.

Elpek KG, Lacelle C, Singh NP, Yolcu ES, Shirwan H (2007) CD4+CD25+ T regulatory cells dominate multiple immune evasion mechanisms in early but not late phases of tumor development in a B cell lymphoma model. *J. Immunol.* 178: 6840-6848.

Escors D, Bricogne C, arce F, Kochan G, Karwacz K (2011) On the mechanism of T cell receptor down-modulation and its physiological significance. *J. Biosci. Med.* 1:pii: 2011.5.

Escors D, Lopes L, Lin R, Hiscott J, Akira S, Davis RJ, Collins MK (2008) Targeting dendritic cell signalling to regulate the response to immunisation. *Blood* 111: 3050-3061.

Fife BT, Pauken KE, Eagar TN, Obu T, Wu J, Tang Q, Azuma M, Krummel MF, Bluestone JA. (2009) Interactions between PD-1 and PD-L1 promote tolerance by blocking the TCR-induced stop signal. *Nat. Immunol.*, Vol. 10, pp. 1185-1192.

Finke JH, Rini B, Ireland J, Rayman P, Richmond A, Golshayan A, Wood L, Elson P, Garcia J, Dreicer R, Bukowski R (2008) Sunitinib reverses type-1 immune suppression and decreases T-regulatory cells in renal cell carcinoma patients. *Clin. Cancer Res.* 14: 6674-6682.

Firat H, Garcia-Pons F, Tourdot S, Pascolo S, Scardino A, Garcia Z, Michel ML, Jack RW, Jung G, Kosmatopoulos K, Mateo L, Suhrbier A, Lemonnier FA, Langlade-Demoyen P (1999) H-2 class I knockout, HLA-A2.1-transgenic mice: a versatile animal model for preclinical evaluation of antitumor immunotherapeutic strategies. *Eur. J. Immunol.* 29: 3112-3121.

Francisco LM, Sage PT, Sharpe AH (2010) The PD-1 pathway in tolerance and autoimmunity. *Immunol. Rev.* 236: 219-242.

Freeman GJ, Long AJ, Iwai Y, Bourque K, Chernova T, Nishimura H, Fitz LJ, Malenkovich N, Okazaki T, Byrne MC, Horton HF, Fouser L, Carter L, Ling V, Bowman MR, Carreno BM, Collins M, Wood CR, Honjo T (2000) Engagement of the PD-1 immunoinhibitory receptor by a novel B7 family member leads to negative regulation of lymphocyte activation. *J. Exp. Med.* 192: 1027-1034.

Ghiringhelli F, Apetoh L, Tesniere A, Aymeric L, Ma Y, Ortiz C, Vermaelen K, Panaretakis T, Mignot G, Ullrich E, Perfettini JL, Schlemmer F, Tasdemir E, Uhl M, Genin P, Civas A, Ryffel B, Kanellopoulos J, Tschopp J, Andre F, Lidereau R, McLaughlin NM, Haynes NM, Smyth MJ, Kroemer G, Zitvogel L (2009) Activation of the NLRP3 inflammasome in dendritic cells induces IL-1beta-dependent adaptive immunity against tumors. *Nat. Med.* 15: 1170-1178.

Goold HD, Escors D, Conlan TJ, Chakraverty R, Bennett CL (2011) Conventional dendritic cells are required for the activation of helper-dependent CD8 T cell responses to a model antigen after cutaneous vaccination with lentiviral vectors. *J. Immunol.* 186: 4565-4572.

Green MR, Monti S, Rodig SJ, Juszczynski P, Currie T, O'Donnell E, Chapuy B, Takeyama K, Neuberg D, Golub TR, Kutok JL, Shipp MA (2010) Integrative analysis reveals selective 9p24.1 amplification, increased PD-1 ligand expression, and further induction via JAK2 in nodular sclerosing Hodgkin lymphoma and primary mediastinal large B-cell lymphoma. *Blood* 116: 3268-3277.

Hansen AK, Regner M, Bonefeld CM, Boding L, Kongsbak M, Odum N, Mullbacher A, Geisler C, von Essen MR (2011) TCR down-regulation boosts T-cell-mediated cytotoxicity and protection against poxvirus infections. *Eur. J. Immunol.* 41: 1948-1957.

He Y, Zhang J, Mi Z, Robbins P, Falo LD, Jr. (2005) Immunization with lentiviral vector-transduced dendritic cells induces strong and long-lasting T cell responses and therapeutic immunity. *J. Immunol.* 174: 3808-3817.

Homann D, Teyton L, Oldstone MB (2001) Differential regulation of antiviral T-cell immunity results in stable CD8+ but declining CD4+ T-cell memory. *Nat. Med.* 7: 913-919.

Kalinski P, Hilkens CM, Wierenga EA, Kapsenberg ML (1999) T-cell priming by type-1 and type-2 polarized dendritic cells: the concept of a third signal. *Immunol Today* 20: 561-567.

Karwacz K, Arce F, Bricogne C, Kochan G, Escors D (2012) PD-L1 co-stimulation, ligand-induced TCR down-modulation and anti-tumor immunotherapy. *Oncoimmunology* 1: 86-88.

Karwacz K, Bricogne C, Macdonald D, Arce F, Bennett CL, Collins M, Escors D (2011) PD-L1 co-stimulation contributes to ligand-induced T cell receptor down-modulation on CD8(+) T cells. *EMBO molecular medicine* 3: 581-592.

Kozako T, Yoshimitsu M, Akimoto M, White Y, Matsushita K, Soeda S, Shimeno H, Kubota R, Izumo S, Arima N (2011) Programmed death-1 (PD-1)/PD-1 ligand pathway-mediated immune responses against human T-lymphotropic virus type 1 (HTLV-1) in HTLV-1-associated myelopathy/tropical spastic paraparesis and carriers with autoimmune disorders. *Human immunology* 72: 1001-1006.

Kozako T, Yoshimitsu M, Fujiwara H, Masamoto I, Horai S, White Y, Akimoto M, Suzuki S, Matsushita K, Uozumi K, Tei C, Arima N (2009) PD-1/PD-L1 expression in human T-cell leukemia virus type 1 carriers and adult T-cell leukemia/lymphoma patients. *Leukemia* 23: 375-382.

Latchman Y, Wood CR, Chernova T, Chaudhary D, Borde M, Chernova I, Iwai Y, Long AJ, Brown JA, Nunes R, Greenfield EA, Bourque K, Boussiotis VA, Carter LL, Carreno BM, Malenkovich N, Nishimura H, Okazaki T, Honjo T, Sharpe AH, Freeman GJ (2001) PD-L2 is a second ligand for PD-1 and inhibits T cell activation. *Nat. Immunol.* 2: 261-268.

Latchman YE, Liang SC, Wu Y, Chernova T, Sobel RA, Klemm M, Kuchroo VK, Freeman GJ, Sharpe AH (2004) PD-L1-deficient mice show that PD-L1 on T cells, antigen-presenting cells, and host tissues negatively regulates T cells. *Proc. Natl. Acad. Sci. USA* 101: 10691-10696.

Liu H, Rhodes M, Wiest DL, Vignali DA (2000) On the dynamics of TCR:CD3 complex cell surface expression and downmodulation. *Immunity* 13: 665-675.

Mangsbo SM, Sandin LC, Anger K, Korman AJ, Loskog A, Totterman TH (2010) Enhanced tumor eradication by combining CTLA-4 or PD-1 blockade with CpG therapy. *Journal of immunotherapy* 33: 225-235.

Mannon RB, Kotzin BL, Nataraj C, Ferri K, Roper E, Kurlander RJ, Coffman TM (1998) Downregulation of T cell receptor expression by CD8(+) lymphocytes in kidney allografts. *J. Clin. Invest.* 101: 2517-2527.

Marzec M, Zhang Q, Goradia A, Raghunath PN, Liu X, Paessler M, Wang HY, Wysocka M, Cheng M, Ruggeri BA, Wasik MA (2008) Oncogenic kinase NPM/ALK induces through STAT3 expression of immunosuppressive protein CD274 (PD-L1, B7-H1). *Proc. Natl. Acad. Sci. USA* 105: 20852-20857.

Morgan RA, Dudley ME, Wunderlich JR, Hughes MS, Yang JC, Sherry RM, Royal RE, Topalian SL, Kammula US, Restifo NP, Zheng Z, Nahvi A, de Vries CR, Rogers-Freezer LJ, Mavroukakis SA, Rosenberg SA (2006) Cancer regression in patients after transfer of genetically engineered lymphocytes. *Science* 314: 126-129.

Naramura M, Jang IK, Kole H, Huang F, Haines D, Gu H (2002) c-Cbl and Cbl-b regulate T cell responsiveness by promoting ligand-induced TCR down-modulation. *Nat. Immunol.* 3: 1192-1199.

Nishimura H, Okazaki T, Tanaka Y, Nakatani K, Hara M, Matsumori A, Sasayama S, Mizoguchi A, Hiai H, Minato N, Honjo T (2001) Autoimmune dilated cardiomyopathy in PD-1 receptor-deficient mice. *Science* 291: 319-322.

Nurieva R, Thomas S, Nguyen T, Martin-Orozco N, Wang Y, Kaja MK, Yu XZ, Dong C (2006) T-cell tolerance or function is determined by combinatorial costimulatory signals. *Embo J.* 25: 2623-2633.

Okazaki T, Tanaka Y, Nishio R, Mitsuiye T, Mizoguchi A, Wang J, Ishida M, Hiai H, Matsumori A, Minato N, Honjo T (2003) Autoantibodies against cardiac troponin I are responsible for dilated cardiomyopathy in PD-1-deficient mice. *Nat. Med.* 9: 1477-1483.

Pilon-Thomas S, Mackay A, Vohra N, Mule JJ (2010) Blockade of programmed death ligand 1 enhances the therapeutic efficacy of combination immunotherapy against melanoma. *J. Immunol.* 184: 3442-3449.

Quigley M, Pereyra F, Nilsson B, Porichis F, Fonseca C, Eichbaum Q, Julg B, Jesneck JL, Brosnahan K, Imam S, Russell K, Toth I, Piechocka-Trocha A, Dolfi D, Angelosanto J, Crawford A, Shin H, Kwon DS, Zupkosky J, Francisco L, Freeman GJ, Wherry EJ, Kaufmann DE, Walker BD, Ebert B, Haining WN (2010) Transcriptional analysis of HIV-specific CD8+ T cells shows that PD-1 inhibits T cell function by upregulating BATF. *Nat. Med.* 16: 1147-1151.

Ramanathan S, Dubois S, Chen XL, Leblanc C, Ohashi PS, Ilangumaran S (2011) Exposure to IL-15 and IL-21 enables autoreactive CD8 T cells to respond to weak antigens and cause disease in a mouse model of autoimmune diabetes. *J. Immunol.* 186: 5131-5141.

Ramanathan S, Dubois S, Gagnon J, Leblanc C, Mariathasan S, Ferbeyre G, Rottapel R, Ohashi PS, Ilangumaran S (2010) Regulation of cytokine-driven functional differentiation of CD8 T cells by suppressor of cytokine signaling 1 controls autoimmunity and preserves their proliferative capacity toward foreign antigens. *J. Immunol.* 185: 357-366.

Sakuishi K, Apetoh L, Sullivan JM, Blazar BR, Kuchroo VK, Anderson AC (2010) Targeting Tim-3 and PD-1 pathways to reverse T cell exhaustion and restore anti-tumor immunity. *J. Exp. Med.* 207: 2187-2194.

Samimi S, Benoit B, Evans K, Wherry EJ, Showe L, Wysocka M, Rook AH (2010) Increased programmed death-1 expression on CD4+ T cells in cutaneous T-cell lymphoma: implications for immune suppression. *Archives of dermatology* 146: 1382-1388.

San Jose E, Borroto A, Niedergang F, Alcover A, Alarcon B (2000) Triggering the TCR complex causes the downregulation of nonengaged receptors by a signal transduction-dependent mechanism. *Immunity* 12: 161-170.

Sharpe AH, Wherry EJ, Ahmed R, Freeman GJ (2007) The function of programmed cell death 1 and its ligands in regulating autoimmunity and infection. *Nat. Immunol.* 8: 239-245.

Sheppard KA, Fitz LJ, Lee JM, Benander C, George JA, Wooters J, Qiu Y, Jussif JM, Carter LL, Wood CR, Chaudhary D (2004) PD-1 inhibits T-cell receptor induced phosphorylation of the ZAP70/CD3zeta signalosome and downstream signaling to PKCtheta. *FEBS Lett* 574: 37-41.

Stagg J, Loi S, Divisekera U, Ngiow SF, Duret H, Yagita H, Teng MW, Smyth MJ (2011) Anti-ErbB-2 mAb therapy requires type I and II interferons and synergizes with anti-PD-1 or anti-CD137 mAb therapy. *Proceedings of the National Academy of Sciences of the United States of America* 108: 7142-7147.

Valitutti S, Muller S, Cella M, Padovan E, Lanzavecchia A. (1995) Serial triggering of many T-cell receptors by a few peptide-MHC complexes. *Nature*, Vol. 375, pp. 148-151.

Van den Eynde BJ, van der Bruggen P (1997) T cell defined tumor antigens. *Current opinion in immunology* 9: 684-693.

Vezys V, Penaloza-MacMaster P, Barber DL, Ha SJ, Konieczny B, Freeman GJ, Mittler RS, Ahmed R (2011) 4-1BB signaling synergizes with programmed death ligand 1 blockade to augment CD8 T cell responses during chronic viral infection. *Journal of immunology* 187: 1634-1642.

Wang J, Yoshida T, Nakaki F, Hiai H, Okazaki T, Honjo T (2005) Establishment of NOD-Pdcd1-/- mice as an efficient animal model of type I diabetes. *Proceedings of the National Academy of Sciences of the United States of America* 102: 11823-11828.

Wang L, Pino-Lagos K, de Vries VC, Guleria I, Sayegh MH, Noelle RJ (2008) Programmed death 1 ligand signaling regulates the generation of adaptive Foxp3+CD4+ regulatory T cells. *Proc. Natl. Acad. Sci. USA* 105: 9331-9336.

Wilcox RA, Feldman AL, Wada DA, Yang ZZ, Comfere NI, Dong H, Kwon ED, Novak AJ, Markovic SN, Pittelkow MR, Witzig TE, Ansell SM (2009) B7-H1 (PD-L1, CD274) suppresses host immunity in T-cell lymphoproliferative disorders. *Blood* 114: 2149-2158.

Xin H, Zhang C, Herrmann A, Du Y, Figlin R, Yu H (2009) Sunitinib inhibition of Stat3 induces renal cell carcinoma tumor cell apoptosis and reduces immunosuppressive cells. *Cancer Res.* 69: 2506-2513.

Zhang L, Gajewski TF, Kline J (2009) PD-1/PD-L1 interactions inhibit antitumor immune responses in a murine acute myeloid leukemia model. *Blood* 114: 1545-1552.

Zitvogel L, Apetoh L, Ghiringhelli F, Kroemer G (2008) Immunological aspects of cancer chemotherapy. *Nature reviews* 8: 59-73.

Reviewed by:

Professor Luis Enjuanes. Email: lenjuanes@cnb.csic.es; Department of Molecular and Cellular Biology, National Centre for Biotechnology (CNB), CSIC, Campus Cantoblanco, 28049 Madrid, Spain.

In: Hodgkin's and T-Cell Lymphoma
Editors: Warren K. Harvey and Randall M. Jacobs
ISBN 978-1-62257-478-0

Chapter 7

COMBINED MODALITY THERAPY IN HODGKIN LYMPHOMA- SHORT TERM BENEFITS AND LONG TERM TOXICITIES- IS THERE EVIDENCE TO DE-ESCALATE THERAPY?

Waleed Khalaf and Nishitha Reddy*
Division of Hematology/Oncology, Department of Medicine,
Vanderbilt University Medical Center, Nashville, TN, US

ABSTRACT

Advances in the treatment of Hodgkin lymphoma (HL) led to improvement in survival outcomes. This success however, brought new challenges in dealing with long-term morbidity. The combined chemotherapy and radiation therapy (CMT) undoubtedly changed the cure rate in this once incurable disease. This approach is associated with long-term toxicities including secondary malignancies and early cardiovascular disease. This led to the launch of many trials investigating the minimal effective therapy that would reduce late toxicities without jeopardizing overall survival. Although an optimal risk stratification system is still elusive, factors such as molecular markers and interim imaging are emerging as prognostic indicators. Radiation therapy plays an important role in a subset of patients with HL, the challenge remains to identify and risk stratify therapy.

Keywords: Radiation therapy, Hodgkin Lymphoma, long term effects, combined modality treatment

* Corresponding author: Nishitha Reddy MD MSCI. Vanderbilt University Medical Center, Nashville, TN 37232; Phone # 615-936-0381; Fax #615-936-8422; Nishitha.reddy@ vanderbilt.edu.

Introduction

Over the past few decades, radiation therapy, either alone or in combination with chemotherapy, has been the key modality for curative treatment of HL achieving cure rates in excess of 80%. Late toxicities from radiation therapy are recognized in long term survivors [1]. HL has a high incidence in children and young adults. Based on the SEER data from 2004 to 2008, the median age at diagnosis was 38 years. Thus, the need to reduce long term treatment effects in survivors, without compromising efficacy of treatment, is of paramount importance. We have certainly seen a paradigm shift over the years in the treatment of HL in an attempt to reduce treatment related toxicities, perhaps none larger than the shift from an extended field radiation to a smaller involved nodal field with reduced total dose delivered. The intriguing question yet remains to be answered if we can possibly select the subgroup that would benefit most with either dose and therapy de-escalation or escalation.

Historical Perspective: Establishment of Combined Modality Approach as the Standard of Care

The first effective use of radiation therapy in HL was reported in 1902, a few years after Roentgen discovered X-rays by Dr. Pusey [2]. The use of Roentgen treatment became the standard approach for HL for the next few decades. In 1931, Rene Gilbert, a Swiss radiologist, published a seminal paper describing his method for extending the field of treatment for HL [3]. Extended field radiation treatment included all clinically involved lymph nodes in a given region as well as all adjacent nodal groups. Evidence for clinical benefit of extending the field of radiation was first presented by Dr. Kaplan in 1962, where more than 70% of the patients treated with extended field radiation were free of disease, whereas those patients treated with a less extended approach had disease recurrence in less than 4 years [4].

The first beneficial use of cytotoxic chemotherapy in HL was reported in 1946 with the use of nitrogen mustard, around the time of World War II while it was being studied as a biological agent for warfare [(5)]. This was followed by a number of reports that confirmed the positive effects of nitrogen mustard either alone, or in combination with radiation therapy. It did not take long until the MOPP combination regimen (nitrogen mustard, vincristine, prednisone, and procarbazine) was developed and was shown to be a superior regimen in advanced stage HL, achieving an initial complete response rate (CR) of 80% and a durable CR in 60% of patients at 3 years [6, 7]. Thereafter, several trials were launched to study the use of CMT using radiation therapy plus MOPP [8]. In the Stanford experience, addition of MOPP to extended field of radiation in early stage disease significantly improved the rate of freedom from relapse, but did not affect the overall survival.

COMPARING CHEMOTHERAPY ALONE TO COMBINED MODALITY THERAPY IN EARLY STAGE, NON-BULKY DISEASE

While interpreting data in HL therapeutic trials one should consider two important aspects: First, the effectiveness of specific treatments such as disease free interval and progression free survival (PFS) and second, the long-term outcomes of the treatment chosen which in turn affects the overall survival (OS). There have been a few randomized trials evaluating the effectiveness of chemotherapy alone compared with CMT (Table 1). In a study at Memorial Sloan-Kettering Cancer Center, 152 untreated patients with clinical stages I to IIIA without bulky disease were randomized between 1990 to 2000 to receive 6 cycles of doxorubicin, bleomycin, vinblastine, and dacarbazine (ABVD) alone or to receive 6 cycles of ABVD followed by 36Gy of radiation therapy (majority received modified extended field radiation). The rate of CR was the same (94% in both groups). At 5 years, 91% of the patients in the CMT group remained in CR as compared with 87% in the ABVD alone arm, but this was not statistically significant. OS at 5 years was 97% for the ABVD plus radiation arm vs. 90% for the ABVD arm, again without reaching statistical significance. Thus, this study could not establish the superiority of addition of radiation therapy to chemotherapy [9].

Table 1. Prospective randomized trials comparing chemotherapy alone to combined chemotherapy plus radiation

Study	# of pts	Chemotherapy	Radiation Dose	PFS (%; CT vs CMT)	OS (%; CT vs CMT)
Straus et al. 2004	152	ABVD x 6 cycles	36 Gy	81 vs 86	90 vs 97
Laskar et al. 2004	179	ABVD x 6 cycles	20-44Gy	94 vs 97	98 vs 100
Nachman et al. 2002	501	COPP/ABV x 4-6 cycles[a]	21 Gy	87 vs 92	98 vs 99
GELA-EORTC H9 trial	619	EBVP x 6 cycle	no XRT vs.20 vs 36 Gy	70 vs 84 vs 87 *	98 vs.96 vs.100
Meyer et al. 2005	399	ABVD x 4-6 cycles	35 Gy	87 vs 93 *	94 vs 96
Meyer et al. 2012	399	ABVD x 4-6 cycles	35 Gy	87 vs 92	94 vs 87% *
Aviles et al. 1998	307	ABVD x 6 cycles	35 Gy	48 vs 78 *	59 vs 88 *

[a] Stage IV patients received intensive combination chemotherapy; CT (chemotherapy), CMT (combined modality treatment), PFS (progression free survival), OS (overall survival), ABVD (doxorubicin, bleomycin, vinblastine, dacarbazine), COPP/ABV (cyclophosphamide, vincristine, procarbazine, prednisone, doxorubicin, bleomycin, vinblastine), EBVP (epirubicin, bleomycin, vinblastine, prednisone); * $P < 0.05$.

Laskar et al. evaluated the role of radiation therapy, mostly involved field radiation, after achieving CR with 6 cycles of ABVD in patients with all stages of HL. Of 251 patients who received ABVD, 179 (71%) achieved CR, and were randomized to receive radiation therapy or no further therapy. In this study, there was an overall significant difference in event-free survival (EFS) and OS in favor of radiation therapy after ABVD at a median follow up of 63 months, however, there was no significant difference in overall outcome, EFS was 94% vs. 97%; OS was 98% vs. 100% for ABVD vs. ABVD plus radiation, respectively [10]. A similarly designed randomized trial from the Children's Cancer Group examining the role of radiation therapy after achieving CR with chemotherapy alone was also reported [11]. In this study, a total of 829 children and adolescents were enrolled between 1995 and 1998. Of those, 501 patients achieved CR and were randomized to receive low dose involved field radiation with 21 Gy or no further therapy. Based on an intent-to-treat analysis, the 3-year EFS was 92% for the group that received radiation as compared with 87% for patients with no further treatment, a difference that was not statistically significant. OS was not significantly different between the two groups, either. These two studies perhaps give us a framework to select patients with early stage disease who may not need radiation therapy, i.e. patients who achieve CR after treatment with chemotherapy alone.

A fourth large trial conducted in collaboration between the National Cancer Institute of Canada and the Eastern Cooperative Oncology Group also addressed the role of chemotherapy alone in early stage HL. In this trial, patients with early non bulky stage I to IIA disease were randomized to either chemotherapy alone with ABVD or CMT. In the arm with ABVD alone, patients received either 4 or 6 total cycles depending on whether they achieved complete remission after the second cycle. In the arm that included radiation treatment, patients received subtotal nodal radiation alone, unless one of the following was present: erythrocyte sedimentation rate ≥ 50mm/h, or four or more nodal sites were involved, in which case those patients were defined as an unfavorable group and thus received 2 cycles of ABVD plus radiation. Approximately, 70% of the patients had one or two unfavorable features, and thus this study was in large part a comparison between combined modality therapy (ABVD x 2 cycles plus radiation) and chemotherapy alone (ABVD x 4-6 cycles). At a median follow up of 4.2 years, the estimated 5-year PFS was 93% for patients who received radiation therapy vs. 87% for patients receiving chemotherapy alone, the only difference that was statistically significant in this study. There was no statistically significant difference in the EFS (88% vs. 86%) or OS (94% vs. 96%) in the group that received ABVD alone or CMT, respectively. In a subset analysis the benefit in PFS with CMT was derived from the unfavorable cohort. The EFS and OS however, were not significantly different when using chemotherapy alone even in this unfavorable cohort [12].

The 12 year follow up of this study was recently reported. The rate of OS was higher in the ABVD only group as compared with the radiation therapy group (94% vs 87%; P=0.04), while the PFS was lower (87% vs. 92%; P=0.05). Interestingly, the OS curve starts to separate between the two groups after ~ 5 years of follow up, which is the typical median follow up time in most clinical trials. As in the case of the reported interim analysis, the difference in the outcomes between the two groups was driven by the differences between the unfavorable risk groups, while there were no significant differences detected in any outcome among patients with favorable risk profile. In terms of cause of death, there were more deaths from causes other than disease relapse in the radiation therapy group as compared with ABVD-only group, including death due to secondary malignancies. Perhaps as telling was the finding of a higher rate of second cancers in general, as well as increased cardiac events in the radiation treatment group. One major criticism of this study that was addressed by the authors is the fact that subtotal nodal radiation is no longer used, and the extent of radiation that was used in this outdated modality very likely contributed to the excess deaths. The curative potential of ABVD alone with a 12-year PFS of 87% and OS of 94% stands alone, making it a viable therapeutic option for those patients. Further, those numbers are even more impressive when a CR is achieved after 2 cycles of ABVD (12-year PFS of 94% and OS of 98%) highlighting the prognostic significance of achieving early CR [13].

Finally, the GELA-EORTC H9 trial randomized early stage HL patients to EBVP (epirubicin, bleomycin, vinblastine and prednisone) chemotherapy alone or in combination with two different radiation doses (20Gy vs. 36 Gy). The 5-year failure free survival was inferior in the EBVP alone arm at 70% compared with 86% and 89% in the 20Gy and 36 Gy radiation arms respectively. This difference was likely due to the inferior chemotherapy regimen that was used. Similar to all the above studies, there was no difference in the overall survival [14].

A number of non-randomized controlled studies have demonstrated similar results with the use of chemotherapy alone in early stage HD. In a prospective trial from Spain, 80 patients with stage I and II non bulky disease who were treated with 6 cycles of ABVD had a PFS of 87% and OS of 97% after a median follow up of 78 months [15]. Another retrospective study from Italy analyzed 139 patients treated with either ABVD alone or CMT between 1995 and 2007 and found similar PFS (83% vs. 80%) and OS (97% vs. 96%) between the two groups [16]. However, 42% of the patients in the combined modality treatment did not receive ABVD, rather, they were treated with the Stanford V regimen, which makes the comparison between the two groups inconclusive. Finally, a recent retrospective study of 75 patients treated with chemotherapy alone at the Dana-Farber Cancer Institute between 1992 and 2008 mostly with 6 cycles of ABVD also demonstrated an excellent outcome using this approach [17]. At a median follow up of at least 50 months, PFS was 92% in the group. At the end of the analysis, no deaths were reported and six patients experienced disease relapse who subsequently achieved CR with salvage therapy that included radiation treatment.

There have also been a few trials showing a benefit of CMT over chemotherapy. A recent meta-analysis pooled the results of five studies that compared chemotherapy alone and CMT [18]. The results of the pooled analysis showed that the addition of radiation therapy significantly improved both OS (HR=0.4; 95% CI 0.27 to 0.61) as well as disease control (HR=0.41; 95% CI 0.25 to 0.66). However, in three of the five analyzed trials, the chemotherapy regimens that were used are considered inferior to ABVD. The trial, which weighed the most heavily on the pooled overall survival, is a large trial from Mexico [19] that compared 6 cycles of ABVD to combination therapy with ABVD x 6 cycles plus extended field radiation therapy with 35-38 Gy. In this study, all patients had bulky disease, limiting relevance of the findings to early stage non-bulky disease. Further, the estimated 12-year OS in the chemotherapy alone arm was lower than would be expected at 59%, and the addition of radiation therapy increased the 12-year OS to 88%. Thus, the pooled results of this meta-analysis are inconclusive as it relates to our patient population of early stage non-bulky disease whether to receive ABVD or a combination approach with ABVD and radiation therapy.

Taken together, these studies show a possible small benefit in PFS for the addition of radiation therapy to chemotherapy with ABVD in early stage, non-bulky HL; however, given the improved salvage treatment options for relapsed patients after chemotherapy alone, and the increased morbidity and mortality associated with radiation therapy, this difference in PFS may not be clinically significant. Based on these results, in early stage disease, clinicians frequently opt to reserve radiation for patients who fail to achieve a complete response to initial chemotherapy.

Evidence for Using Radiation in Bulky and Advanced HL

In patients with bulky disease (>10 cm) radiation therapy has been incorporated as part of the treatment regimen- There are no randomized trials comparing chemotherapy alone with CMT.

In a large randomized trial by Hoskin et al., patients with advanced and bulky HL were randomized to ABVD + radiation or Stanford V regimen. The Stanford V regimen incorporates 36 Gy for bulky disease and 30 Gy for sites of non-bulky disease. In the latter half of the study patients were subjected to radiation only if they did not achieve a CR. In this study, approximately 90 patients in each arm had bulky disease. In an exploratory analysis of this study comparing PFS among those who received radiation and those who did not, there was no difference among the patients randomized to the ABVD or Stanford V. There was lower PFS in patients who received Stanford V and no radiation suggesting that patients assigned to Stanford V should receive radiation therapy [20].

In a randomized phase III study comparing 2 different CMT regimens; ABVD + radiation vs. Stanford V regimen, there was no statistically significant differences in either FFS or OS between both the groups [21]. The long term radiation side effects on these trials are unavailable; however, do raise an important question if it is necessary to subject all patients to XRT.

In a different study, patients with previously untreated stage III or IV HL were treated with MOPP- ABV (mechlorethamine, vinblastine, procarbazine, prednisone, doxorubicin, bleomycin and vinblastine) and subsequently randomized to either receive or not receive radiation. Patients who had bulky disease were randomized to either treatment arm if they attained a CR. Patients who achieved a partial response (PR) received radiation and were excluded from being randomized. In this study, pts who received radiation after CR had a higher death rate than did pts who did not receive radiation. The 5-year probability of secondary malignancies in patients who received radiation was twice that of the patients who did not receive radiation. The rate of acute myeloid leukemia (AML) and myelodysplastic syndrome (MDS) were higher among these patients. It can be argued that the chemotherapy regimen included mechlorethamine which is known to alter the stem cells, but that needs further investigation. This study does highlight the fact that all patients with bulky disease may not need to be subjected to radiation therapy [22].

Late Effects of Radiation Therapy

Over the past few decades, it is becoming more apparent that long term survivors of HL are at an increased risk or morbidity and mortality from causes directly related to the exposed treatment.

Cardiovascular Effects

Numerous studies have shown increased cardiac mortality as well as morbidity in long term survivors of HL as compared with the general population [23, 24, 25, 26, 27]. A wide spectrum of cardiac diseases has been reported, including coronary artery disease, valvular disease, pericardial disease, ventricular dysfunction, and conduction abnormalities[28-30]. The estimated relative risk of cardiac mortality ranges from 2.2 to 12.7 and this elevated risk persist 20-30 years after initial treatment [31]. This collection of data captures patients that have been treated with different modalities of radiation and chemotherapy, including historically extended field radiation. A potential contributor to the increased cardiovascular mortality is the cytotoxic chemotherapy, either by itself, or in combination with radiation therapy. However, it is clear that the addition of radiation therapy does increase the risk of cardiovascular mortality in those patients. This was demonstrated in a large study by Boivin et al. [32] where radiation to the mediastinum increased the relative risk (RR) of death from myocardial infarction by 2.6 compared with patients who did not receive mediastinal radiation, and that cardiac mortality was proportionally related to the radiation dose. The increase in RR was not seen in patients who received chemotherapy alone. Indeed, a number of guidelines have been adopted for screening of cardiovascular disease in long term survivors who received radiation as part of their treatment, including published guidelines by Children's Oncology Group (COG), National Comprehensive Cancer Network (NCCN), and American College of Radiology (ACR).

Endocrine Effects

In CMT both men and women are at risk of hypothyroidism and hypogonadism if exposed to supradiaprhagmatic or infradiaphragmatic radiation therapy. Recently with the use of limited field radiation, gonadal-sparing radiation, and modified chemotherapy the risk of hypogonadism may have decreased. Hypothyroidism however continues to be a concern. It is recommended that patients who have been exposed to radiation involving the neck, TSH be checked at least yearly. Further, fertility issues need to be addressed with young patients prior to treatment initiation.

Secondary Malignancies

Patients exposed to CMT are at an increased risk of lung cancer and women are at risk for breast cancer- Other solid tumor malignancies such as GI cancers, sarcomas are also increased. In a cohort of 6647 female survivors of childhood cancer who received radiation therapy a linear increase in breast cancer risk was reported with increasing doses up to 40 Gy[33, 34]. The risk of lung cancer, bone sarcomas and gastrointestinal malignancies also rise with increasing radiation doses and exposed lung volume[35, 36]. An interesting observation that the risk of thyroid cancer decreased with a decrease in the volume of normal tissue radiated suggests that limiting the exposure of normal tissue to radiation doses can reduce the risk of secondary malignancies [37].

Pulmonary Complications

Pulmonary toxicity occurs in patients exposed to pulmonary radiation and/or chemotherapy that include bleomycin. Hypoalbuminemia and the use of colony stimulating factors have been associated with the risk of development of pneumonitis [38]. Combination chemotherapy and radiotherapy was associated with sub-clinical pulmonary toxicity. These patients experienced a decrease in their diffusion capacity and total lung capacity [39].

Taking into consideration, the above toxicities which can lead to significant morbidity, thus, avoiding radiation therapy or limiting the field of radiation in patients who may not derive much benefit from radiation is of paramount importance.

PET and Gene Signatures in Establishing Treatment Plan

Until the development of FDG-PET scan, the international prognostic score (IPS) which includes 7 variables in newly diagnosed HL patients carried prognostic information [40]. Gallamini et al. originally published the results of the value of interim PET scan and its prognostic significance. Among the 260 patients with HL, the 2 year PFS for negative PET after 2 cycles of ABVD was 95% and 13% for those with PET positive scan. The overall sensitivity of an interim PET scan is 81% sensitive and 97% specific [41, 42]. The major controversy that surrounds the prognostic utility of these scans is the interpreter variability. Specific guidelines have been developed namely the Deauville criteria in an attempt to standardize the reading [43]. Therefore, an interim PET scan is of prognostic value and its role in changing early treatment evaluation is the key question that remains unanswered [42].

Using gene expression profiling, Steidl et al. identified a gene signature with tumor macrophages that is predictive of treatment failure. A concurrent immunohistochemical analysis revealed that an increase in the number of CD68+ cells was associated with a poor outcome irrespective of the IPS score. Patients with a higher number of CD68 cells had an inferior PFS of 2.7 years compared with those with low CD68 + cells in whom median survival was not reached [44]. It remains to be elucidated if CD68 and PET imaging can help guide therapy.

Modifications in Radiation Therapy

The HD8 trial resulted in a switch form extended field radiation therapy to involved field radiation after chemotherapy in early unfavorable HL [45]. Involved nodal radiation therapy (INRT) and intensity modulated radiation therapy (IMRT) are interesting emerging concepts to be explored in HL. INRT involves radiating the involved lymph nodes as well as a pre-defined margin, usually less than 5 cm. This was compared with IFRT retrospectively. There was no increase in loco regional relapse by limiting the radiation field [46]. IMRT delivers higher intensity beams to the tumor and lower intensity to the normal tissue which is crucial while radiating the mediastinum [47]. INRT is gaining momentum and is being rapidly incorporated in therapy of HL.

FUTURE CHALLENGES

The new challenges moving forward include identifying patients where treatment may be tailored to include or avoid the addition of radiation therapy. It also remains to be seen what the value of the different new prognostic information is and how those are integrated into making treatment decisions. Based on PET imaging, response adapted therapy is currently being evaluated under clinical trials- in united States and Europe in the hope to answer the question of de-escalating or intensifying chemotherapy in selected individuals thus minimizing long-term toxicities. The mere fact that we are able to discuss treatment reduction and early treatment modification strategies should highlight the successes that have been accomplished in the HL treatment over the past few decades.

REFERENCES

[1] Armitage JO. Early-stage Hodgkin's lymphoma. *N Engl J Med.* 2010 Aug 12;363(7):653-62.

[2] Pusey W. Cases of sarcoma and of Hodgkin's disease treated by exposures to X-rays - A preliminary report. *AMA.* 1902; XXXVIII(3):166-9.

[3] Gilbert R, Babaintz L. Our method of roentgentherapie lymphogranuloma (Hodgkin); Remote results. *Act Radiol.* 1931;12:523-9.

[4] Kaplan HS. The radical radiotherapy of regionally localized Hodgkin's disease. *Radiology.* 1962 Apr;78:553-61.

[5] Gilman A, Philips FS. The biological actions and therapeutic applications of the B-chloroethyl amines and sulfides. *Science.* 1946 Apr 5;103(2675):409-15.

[6] Frei E, 3rd, DeVita VT, Moxley JH, 3rd, Carbone PP. Approaches to improving the chemotherapy of Hodgkin's disease. *Cancer Res.* 1966 Jun;26(6):1284-9.

[7] Devita VT, Jr., Serpick AA, Carbone PP. Combination chemotherapy in the treatment of advanced Hodgkin's disease. *Ann Intern Med* 1970 Dec;73(6):881-95.

[8] Rosenberg SA, Kaplan HS. The management of stages I, II, and III Hodgkin's disease with combined radiotherapy and chemotherapy. *Cancer.* 1975 Jan;35(1):55-63.

[9] Straus DJ, Portlock CS, Qin J, Myers J, Zelenetz AD, Moskowitz C, et al. Results of a prospective randomized clinical trial of doxorubicin, bleomycin, vinblastine, and dacarbazine (ABVD) followed by radiation therapy (RT) versus ABVD alone for stages I, II, and IIIA nonbulky Hodgkin disease. *Blood.* 2004 Dec 1;104(12):3483-9.

[10] Laskar S, Gupta T, Vimal S, Muckaden MA, Saikia TK, Pai SK, et al. Consolidation radiation after complete remission in Hodgkin's disease following six cycles of doxorubicin, bleomycin, vinblastine, and dacarbazine chemotherapy: is there a need? *J Clin Oncol.* 2004 Jan 1;22(1):62-8.

[11] Nachman JB, Sposto R, Herzog P, Gilchrist GS, Wolden SL, Thomson J, et al. Randomized comparison of low-dose involved-field radiotherapy and no radiotherapy for children with Hodgkin's disease who achieve a complete response to chemotherapy. *J Clin Oncol.* 2002 Sep 15;20(18):3765-71.

[12] Meyer RM, Gospodarowicz MK, Connors JM, Pearcey RG, Bezjak A, Wells WA, et al. Randomized comparison of ABVD chemotherapy with a strategy that includes

radiation therapy in patients with limited-stage Hodgkin's lymphoma: National Cancer Institute of Canada Clinical Trials Group and the Eastern Cooperative Oncology Group. *J Clin Oncol.* 2005 Jul 20;23(21):4634-42.

[13] Meyer RM, Gospodarowicz MK, Connors JM, Pearcey RG, Wells WA, Winter JN, et al. ABVD alone versus radiation-based therapy in limited-stage Hodgkin's lymphoma. *N Engl J Med.* 2012 Feb 2;366(5):399-408.

[14] Eghbali H, Brice P, Creemers GY, van Marwijk Kooij M, Carde P, Van't Veer MB, et al. Comparison of three radiation dose levels after EBVP regimen in favorable supradiaphragmatic clinical stages (CS) I-II Hodgkin's lymphoma (HL): Preliminary results of the EORTC-GELA H9-F trial. *Blood* (ASH Annual Meeting Abstracts). 2005;106:814a.

[15] Rueda Dominguez A, Marquez A, Guma J, Llanos M, Herrero J, de Las Nieves MA, et al. Treatment of stage I and II Hodgkin's lymphoma with ABVD chemotherapy: results after 7 years of a prospective study. *Ann Oncol.* 2004 Dec;15(12):1798-804.

[16] Olcese F, Clavio M, Rossi E, Spriano M, Ballerini F, Canepa L, et al. The addition of radiotherapy to chemotherapy does not improve outcome of early stage Hodgkin's lymphoma patients: a retrospective long-term follow-up analysis of a regional Italian experience. *Ann Hematol.* 2009 Sep;88(9):855-61.

[17] Canellos GP, Abramson JS, Fisher DC, LaCasce AS. Treatment of favorable, limited-stage Hodgkin's lymphoma with chemotherapy without consolidation by radiation therapy. *J Clin Oncol.* 2010 Mar 20;28(9):1611-5.

[18] Herbst C, Rehan FA, Skoetz N, Bohlius J, Brillant C, Schulz H, et al. Chemotherapy alone versus chemotherapy plus radiotherapy for early stage Hodgkin lymphoma. *Cochrane Database Syst Rev.* 2011(2):CD007110.

[19] Aviles A, Delgado S. A prospective clinical trial comparing chemotherapy, radiotherapy and combined therapy in the treatment of early stage Hodgkin's disease with bulky disease. *Clin Lab Haematol.* 1998 Apr;20(2):95-9.

[20] Hoskin PJ, Rojas AM, Bentzen SM, Saunders MI. Radiotherapy with concurrent carbogen and nicotinamide in bladder carcinoma. *J Clin Oncol.* 2010 Nov 20;28(33):4912-8.

[21] Advani R, Hong FX, Fisher RI, Bartlett NL, Robinson S, Gascoyne RD, et al. Randomized Phase III Trial Comparing ABVD plus Radiotherapy and the Stanford V.Regimen In Patients with Stage I/II Bulky Mediastinal Hodgkin Lymphoma: A-Subset Analysis of the US Intergroup Trial E2496. *Blood.* 2010 Nov 19;116(21):185-6.

[22] Aleman BM, Raemaekers JM, Tirelli U, Bortolus R, van 't Veer MB, Lybeert ML, et al. Involved-field radiotherapy for advanced Hodgkin's lymphoma. *N Engl J Med.* 2003 Jun 12;348(24):2396-406.

[23] van Rijswijk RE, Verbeek J, Haanen C, Dekker AW, van Daal WA, van Peperzeel HA. Major complications and causes of death in patients treated for Hodgkin's disease. *J Clin Oncol.* 1987 Oct;5(10):1624-33.

[24] Hancock SL, Tucker MA, Hoppe RT. Factors affecting late mortality from heart disease after treatment of Hodgkin's disease. *JAMA.* 1993 Oct 27;270(16):1949-55.

[25] Aleman BM, van den Belt-Dusebout AW, De Bruin ML, van 't Veer MB, Baaijens MH, de Boer JP, et al. Late cardiotoxicity after treatment for Hodgkin lymphoma. *Blood.* 2007 Mar 1;109(5):1878-86.

[26] Swerdlow AJ, Higgins CD, Smith P, Cunningham D, Hancock BW, Horwich A, et al. Myocardial infarction mortality risk after treatment for Hodgkin disease: a collaborative British cohort study. *J Natl Cancer Inst.* 2007 Feb 7;99(3):206-14.

[27] Castellino SM, Geiger AM, Mertens AC, Leisenring WM, Tooze JA, Goodman P, et al. Morbidity and mortality in long-term survivors of Hodgkin lymphoma: a report from the Childhood Cancer Survivor Study. *Blood.* 2011 Feb 10;117(6):1806-16.

[28] Heidenreich PA, Hancock SL, Lee BK, Mariscal CS, Schnittger I. Asymptomatic cardiac disease following mediastinal irradiation. *J Am Coll Cardiol.* 2003 Aug 20;42(4):743-9.

[29] Heidenreich PA, Hancock SL, Vagelos RH, Lee BK, Schnittger I. Diastolic dysfunction after mediastinal irradiation. *Am Heart J.* 2005 Nov;150(5):977-82.

[30] Hull MC, Morris CG, Pepine CJ, Mendenhall NP. Valvular dysfunction and carotid, subclavian, and coronary artery disease in survivors of hodgkin lymphoma treated with radiation therapy. *JAMA.* 2003 Dec 3;290(21):2831-7.

[31] Ng AK. Review of the cardiac long-term effects of therapy for Hodgkin lymphoma. *Br J Haematol.* 2011 Jul;154(1):23-31.

[32] Boivin JF, Hutchison GB, Lubin JH, Mauch P. Coronary artery disease mortality in patients treated for Hodgkin's disease. *Cancer.* 1992 Mar 1;69(5):1241-7.

[33] Inskip PD, Robison LL, Stovall M, Smith SA, Hammond S, Mertens AC, et al. Radiation dose and breast cancer risk in the childhood cancer survivor study. *J Clin Oncol.* 2009 Aug 20;27(24):3901-7.

[34] Travis LB, Hill DA, Dores GM, Gospodarowicz M, van Leeuwen FE, Holowaty E, et al. Breast cancer following radiotherapy and chemotherapy among young women with Hodgkin disease. *JAMA.* 2003 Jul 23;290(4):465-75.

[35] Hawkins MM, Wilson LM, Burton HS, Potok MH, Winter DL, Marsden HB, et al. Radiotherapy, alkylating agents, and risk of bone cancer after childhood cancer. *J Natl Cancer Inst.* 1996 Mar 6;88(5):270-8.

[36] van den Belt-Dusebout AW, Aleman BM, Besseling G, de Bruin ML, Hauptmann M, van 't Veer MB, et al. Roles of radiation dose and chemotherapy in the etiology of stomach cancer as a second malignancy. *Int J Radiat Oncol Biol Phys.* 2009 Dec 1;75(5):1420-9.

[37] Sigurdson AJ, Ronckers CM, Mertens AC, Stovall M, Smith SA, Liu Y, et al. Primary thyroid cancer after a first tumour in childhood (the Childhood Cancer Survivor Study): a nested case-control study. *Lancet.* 2005 Jun 11-17;365(9476):2014-23.

[38] Ngeow J, Tan IB, Kanesvaran R, Tan HC, Tao M, Quek R, et al. Prognostic impact of bleomycin-induced pneumonitis on the outcome of Hodgkin's lymphoma. *Ann Hematol.* 2011 Jan;90(1):67-72.

[39] Villani F, Busia A, Villani M, Laffranchi A, Viviani S, Bonfante V. Cardiopulmonary response to exercise in patients with different degrees of lung toxicity after radio-chemotherapy for Hodgkin's disease. *Anticancer Res.* 2009 Feb;29(2):777-83.

[40] Hasenclever D, Diehl V. A prognostic score for advanced Hodgkin's disease. International Prognostic Factors Project on Advanced Hodgkin's Disease. *N Engl J Med.* 1998 Nov 19;339(21):1506-14.

[41] Gallamini A, Hutchings M, Rigacci L, Specht L, Merli F, Hansen M, et al. Early interim 2-[18F]fluoro-2-deoxy-D-glucose positron emission tomography is prognostically superior to international prognostic score in advanced-stage Hodgkin's

lymphoma: a report from a joint Italian-Danish study. *J Clin Oncol.* 2007 Aug 20;25(24):3746-52.

[42] Terasawa T, Lau J, Bardet S, Couturier O, Hotta T, Hutchings M, et al. Fluorine-18-fluorodeoxyglucose positron emission tomography for interim response assessment of advanced-stage Hodgkin's lymphoma and diffuse large B-cell lymphoma: a systematic review. *J Clin Oncol.* 2009 Apr 10;27(11):1906-14.

[43] Barrington SF, Qian W, Somer EJ, Franceschetto A, Bagni B, Brun E, et al. Concordance between four European centres of PET reporting criteria designed for use in multicentre trials in Hodgkin lymphoma. Eur *J Nucl Med Mol Imaging.* 2010 Oct;37(10):1824-33.

[44] Steidl C, Lee T, Shah SP, Farinha P, Han G, Nayar T, et al. Tumor-associated macrophages and survival in classic Hodgkin's lymphoma. *N Engl J Med.* 2010 Mar 11;362(10):875-85.

[45] Engert A, Schiller P, Josting A, Herrmann R, Koch P, Sieber M, et al. Involved-field radiotherapy is equally effective and less toxic compared with extended-field radiotherapy after four cycles of chemotherapy in patients with early-stage unfavorable Hodgkin's lymphoma: results of the HD8 trial of the German Hodgkin's Lymphoma Study Group. *J Clin Oncol.* 2003 Oct 1;21(19):3601-8.

[46] Campbell BA, Voss N, Pickles T, Morris J, Gascoyne RD, Savage KJ, et al. Involved-nodal radiation therapy as a component of combination therapy for limited-stage Hodgkin's lymphoma: a question of field size. *J Clin Oncol.* 2008 Nov 10;26(32):5170-4.

[47] Chera BS, Rodriguez C, Morris CG, Louis D, Yeung D, Li Z, et al. Dosimetric comparison of three different involved nodal irradiation techniques for stage II Hodgkin's lymphoma patients: conventional radiotherapy, intensity-modulated radiotherapy, and three-dimensional proton radiotherapy. *Int J Radiat Oncol Biol Phys.* 2009 Nov 15;75(4):1173-80.

In: Hodgkin's and T-Cell Lymphoma
Editors: Warren K. Harvey and Randall M. Jacobs
ISBN 978-1-62257-478-0

Chapter 8

ENTEROPATHY-ASSOCIATED T-CELL LYMPHOMA

Kevin McDonnell and Ryan Wilcox
University of Michigan, Division of Hematology
and Oncology, Ann Arbor, MI, US

ABSTRACT

Enteropathy–Associated T-Cell Lymphoma (EATL) is an extranodal peripheral T-cell lymphoma derived from intraepithelial lymphocytes (IELs) of the intestinal mucosa that commonly involves the small intestine and is classically associated with celiac sprue. EATLs, classified by the World Health Organization (WHO) into two subtypes with distinct clinical and pathologic features, are aggressive lymphomas with a dismal prognosis. Disease- and treatment-related complications, along with chemorefractory disease, are common. Therefore, the median overall survival is less than one year, with few long-term survivors. Improved understanding of the molecular pathogenesis of EATL is greatly needed if novel therapeutic approaches are to be developed for this aggressive and poorly understood T-cell lymphoma. In this chapter we will review the natural history, diagnosis, risk-stratification, and treatment strategies for EATL.

I. INTRODUCTION

EATL is an extranodal peripheral T-cell lymphoma characterized by the infiltration and expansion of malignant T-cells within the intestinal epithelium, most commonly the small intestine [1]. EATL is rare, representing less than 10% of all peripheral T-cell lymphomas (PTCLs). The WHO has identified two subcategories of EATL, type 1 and type 2. Type 1 EATL, strongly associated with celiac disease (CD) and more common in Europe, frequently evolves from clonally expanded IELs. In contrast, type 2 EATL is less commonly associated with CD and represents the majority of EATL cases in Asia [2]. Anthracycline-based chemotherapy is frequently employed in the management of EATL and is associated with improved, yet disappointing, disease-free and overall survivals [3]. Future investigations may yield an improved understanding of EATL pathogenesis and lead to the development of novel therapeutic strategies.

II. Classification and Epidemiology

EATL is a rare but increasingly prevalent non-Hodgkin lymphoma with a current annual incidence of approximately 0.75 per million [3-5]. The median age of onset of EATL is in the sixth decade [6]. Originally recognized as a CD-associated lymphoma in the mid twentieth century, EATL remains the most common cancer in patients with CD, particularly those with refractory disease [7-9]. In 2008, the WHO recognized two EATL subtypes that are histologically and genetically distinct [10-16].

The histology of type 1 EATL is characterized by medium to large cells with irregular nuclear contours within a background of reactive eosinophils, histiocytes, and small lymphocytes [17-21]. Consistent with its frequent association with CD, EATL type 1 is often detected within the context of ongoing intestinal mucosal tissue inflammation with intestinal crypt hyperplasia and villous atrophy [12, 22]. In contrast, type 2 EATL is characterized by monomorphic small- to medium-sized cells with round or oval nuclei and stippled chromatin [23-25]. Type 1 EATL occurs more frequently among populations noted to have a high incidence of CD, including those with the HLA-DQ2 and HLA-DQ8 haplotypes [3]. Individuals with these genotypes more commonly originate from Western and Northern European populations [23, 26, 27]. Conversely, Type 2 EATL is more frequently observed in non HLA-DQ2 and HLA-DQ8 expressing Asian populations [11, 28-31]. Recently, the International Peripheral T-Cell Lymphoma Project confirmed the geographic and population differences characteristic of these EATL subtypes [3]. Clonal T-cells in EATL type 1 are CD3+, CD4-, and CD8-/+, and commonly express perforin, granzyme B, or TIA-1, suggesting their derivation from cytotoxic IELs. CD30 is more commonly expressed in type 1 than in type 2 EATL, and CD56 is usually expressed in type 2EATL, but is present in only a minority of type 1 cases.

Genetically, both type 1 and type 2 EATLs frequently exhibit 9q31.3 amplifications and deletions of 16q12.1. Compared with type 2 EATL, type 1 EATL more frequently demonstrates gains in chromosomes 1q and 5q. Amplification of 8q24 (MYC) is apparently unique to type 2 EATL [10, 11, 13, 32].

The incidence of CD is rising worldwide in populations with a historically elevated incidence of CD, and in populations within Latin America, North Africa and the Middle East that are not traditionally associated with CD [33-36]. The rising incidence of CD has translated into increased risk for the development of type 1 EATL [6]. Multiple factors may be contributing to this increase in CD and type 1 EATL including, among others, a global increase in the consumption of wheat and gluten products as well as the selective breeding and/or genetic engineering of wheat strains which has increased the gluten content of cereal crops [37-41].

III. PATHOGENESIS

EATL evolves from clonally expanded intraepithelial *alpha/beta* T-cells.The association between EATL and CD has been strengthened recently by both genetic and immunologic investigations elucidating the immune processing and reactivity of gluten peptides [10]. The pathogenesis of CD is initiated with the translocation of gluten peptides (derived from digested wheat, barley or rye) through a compromised intestinal epithelium that may occur secondary to infection or other inflammatory insults [42]. Upon traversing the epithelium, gluten peptides are deamidated via the enzymatic action of tissue transglutaminase, thereby augmenting their antigenicity when presented by specific HLA class II molecules expressed on professional antigen-presenting cells within the gut. With initiation of a T-cell response, cytokine production culminates in tissue damage, leading to villous atrophy and crypt hyperplasia. Evidence is emerging that cytokines, such IL-15, are important in CD pathogenesis and contribute to the growth and survival of malignant T cells in EATL [43].

By adopting a gluten free diet and eliminating exposure to antigenic gluten-derived peptides, patients may alleviate their symptoms of CD, reestablish a normal small intestinal cytoarchitecture and reduce their risk of developing EATL. A minority of patients, despite adhering to a gluten-free diet, does not achieve complete histologic or clinical resolution of CD [44, 45]. These patients with so-called refractory CD (RCD) remain at particularly high risk of progression to type 1 EATL, especially when associated with phenotypically abnormal IELs [18, 46].

In addition to the influence that HLA genetics have upon the development of CD and type 1 EATL, additional genetic determinants have been identified. Non-HLA genes which may contribute to the development of CD and type 1 EATL include myosin IXB (MYO9B), located on chromosome 19. The MYO9B gene product is a myosin molecule expressed in the epithelial cells of the gastrointestinal tract [47]. Variants in the MYO9B gene product may alter the physical integrity of the intestinal mucosa permitting increased passage of antigens across the gastrointestinal epithelium. [48]. In addition to the chromosome 19 MYO9B locus, other loci have been identified in genetic linkage studies, implicating genes on chromosomes 5, 6, 9 and15 [49][50][59].

Compared with type 1 EATL, the pathogenesis underlying type 2 EATL remains less well described. Although type 1 and type 2 EATLs share a similar cell of origin, the oncogenic pathways exploited by type 2 EATL may be distinct. In contrast to type 1 EATL, the chronic antigenic, inflammatory or molecular stimuli that may promote type 2 EATL pathogenesis remain incompletely described. Recent investigations documenting novel molecular pathways operative in intestinal intraepithelial lymphocytes may provide insights into the etiology of type 2 EATL. Gene amplifications of c-Myc, which genetically distinguish type 1 from type 2 EATL, may upregulate expression of the IL-15 receptor [51]. This may increase sensitivity to IL-15-mediated anti-apoptotic signaling, thus contributing to the malignant transformation of IELs. Further investigations into the molecular pathways governing the biology of the IEL will be required for complete delineation of the pathogenesis of type 2 EATL.

IV. Clinical Characteristics, Diagnosis and Risk Stratification

EATL characteristically is diagnosed at an advanced-stage and is clinically aggressive. Not surprisingly, patients frequently present with abdominal-related complaints - pain, perforation, obstruction, bleeding, and anorexia. In addition, B symptoms and fatigue are common. In Type 1 EATL, escalation of CD-related symptoms frequently heralds the development of EATL; in type 2 EATL precedent CD-related symptoms are rare. Characteristically, the clinical course of EATL is rapidly progressive with survival measured in months [2, 3, 14, 17, 25, 29, 52-57].

The recommended initial assessment of EATL follows that normally performed for any peripheral T-cell lymphoma including histological assessment, immunophenotyping, and cytogenetics of a tissue specimen together with a history and physical examination with basic laboratory assessment. Imaging studies, including PET/CT, are typically performed. A bone marrow biopsy is also recommended, although bone marrow involvement is rare. Endoscopic assessment of the gastrointestinal tract is useful for obtaining tissue and assessing the extent of small bowel involvement [58]. A number of novel imaging techniques have been used in the evaluation of EATL in order to provide enhanced diagnostic assessment of the patient with EATL. For example, magnetic resonance imaging of the bowel provides enhanced sensitivity for detection of primary disease as well as assessing response to therapy [59, 60].

Double balloon enteroscopy is another imaging approach proving to be a valuable diagnostic tool in the assessment of EATL as it permits both the direct visualization of the gastrointestinal tract and the securing of tissue specimens for pathologic assessment [61-63].

Other novel gastrointestinal imaging modalities such as confocal endomicroscopy and molecular imaging techniques may also prove to be valuable diagnostic modalities in the evaluation of EATL [64, 65].

The initial assessment of EATL allows determination of disease stage. The Ann Arbor Staging system is most frequently employed to define the extent of disease in EATL [3, 58], though some advocate the use of alternative staging schemas, including the 1994 Gastrointestinal Tract Lymphoma Workshop staging system [2, 66].

A variety of prognostic scoring systems have been employed to risk-stratify patients with EATL, including the International Prognostic Index (IPI) and the Prognostic Index for Peripheral T-Cell Lymphoma (PIT) [67, 68]. The IPI employs the parameters of age, performance status, lactate dehydrogenase (LDH) values, the presence of extranodal involvement, and Ann Arbor stage, to estimate outcome. In comparison, the PIT relies on age, performance status, LDH values and the presence of bone marrow involvement. The International Peripheral T-Cell Lymphoma Project has demonstrated that the PIT outperforms the IPI with regard to prediction of overall and failure-free survival [3]. The variables included in the PIT are more relevant in EATL, and likely explain its superiority to the IPI in risk-stratifying patients with EATL. The International Peripheral T-Cell Lymphoma Project additionally demonstrated that tumor size (≥5 cm.) and an elevated C-reactive protein were adverse prognostic factors.

The use of an anthracycline-containing chemotherapy regimen was also associated with improved survival. Other variables typically of prognostic utility in non-Hodgkin's lymphomas, such as the proliferative index and Ann Arbor stage, were not found to have prognostic significance.

Furthermore, no difference in survival between patients with type 1 EATL and type 2 EATL was observed. The utility of prognostic scoring systems currently available for EATL is limited by the overall poor outcome of these patients. This limitation reflects the lack of effective therapeutic options in EATL and highlights the need for the development of improved treatment approaches.

VI. Treatment

Studies investigating the efficacy and outcomes of treatments for EATL are limited by its low incidence. Furthermore, the high morbidity/mortality of EATL at the time of diagnosis and poor performance status observed in many patients limit their ability to tolerate multiagent chemotherapeutic regimens [3, 55].

A variety of treatments are employed for EATL. Initial therapy for EATL may include immediate surgical intervention in up to one half of patients to address a serious life-threatening gastrointestinal complication such as bowel perforation or to alleviate an intestinal obstruction [53, 69, 70]. Overall, superior outcomes are achieved with complete resection of disease at time of surgical intervention compared with partial resection [2, 55, 71, 72]. Radiation therapy is only rarely employed and most typically implemented to achieve palliative debulking of an obstructing lesion prior to beginning other treatments [53].

Unfortunately, the majority of patients cannot receive multiagent chemotherapy due to a poor or declining performance states [17]. For those EATL patients able to initiate therapy, multiagent, anthracycline-based regimens (e.g. CHOP) are generally employed and have been shown to be superior to non-anthracycline containing regimens [3, 58]. The most utilized first-line regimen for the treatment of EATL is CHOP,with or without the addition of other agents such as etoposide (CHOEP). An alternate regimen is HyperCVAD with high-dose methotrexate and cytarabine. Other anthracycline-based regimenshave been reported [52, 70, 72]. With these regimens, overall response rates of between 50 and 60% and 5 year survivals of 20-25% have been observed [3, 52, 73]. Second line therapies, as for other non-Hodgkin lymphomas, include ICE and DHAP, although FC (fludarabine, cyclophosphamide) and cladribine have been used [71]. Unfortunately, durable remissions are seldom attained. Remission rates are disappointing with only about 40% of patients achieving a complete response following first-line treatment with an anthracycline-based regimen. Overall survival remains dismal, with median overall survival of less than 12 months, and long-term survival is rare [3, 17, 52, 70, 74, 75].

High-dose chemotherapy and autologous stem-cell transplantation (HDT/ASCT) has been used in an attempt to improve survival in EATL [76]. As with the use of systemic chemotherapy, the poor performance status, rapid progression, and frequency of chemorefractory disease preclude this approach for many patients. For carefully selected cohorts of patients, novel regimens followed by HDT/ASCT may provide clinical benefit. For example, the use of CHOP followed by IVE (ifosfamide, epirubicin, etoposide)/intermediate-dose methotrexate followed by HDT/ASCT has recently been demonstrated to achieve a five year progression-free and overall survival of 52% and 60% respectively, which is superior to the historical results achieved with traditional anthracycline-based regimens [75]. Additional transplantation regimens have been used with variable success [77][78][75, 79-82].

A variety of innovative therapies for EATL have been instituted with the intent of improving response rates and survival outcomes. Prominent among these therapies is the use of the anti-CD52 monoclonal antibody alemtuzumab. In one recent study involving patients with peripheral T-cell lymphomas, including EATL, CHOP combined with alemtuzumab was associated with a complete response rate of 71% and an overall median duration of response of 11 months [83]. Other studies using alemtuzumab have had mixed results [84, 85]. Additional investigational agents for use in the treatment of EATL are being explored, including the use of antibodies to target IL-15 and histone deacetylase inhibitors [43, 86].

CONCLUSION

EATL is a rare extranodal peripheral T-cell lymphoma. Its prevalence is increasing along with the overall global increase in CD. EATL remains a morbid PTCL, often presenting with life-threatening complications, including intestinal perforation and sepsis. Current treatments, including anthracycline-based regimens, yield disappointing results with a median overall survival less than 12 months. Novel multiagent regimens followed by HDT/ASCT may be associated with improved outcomes for appropriately selected patients. Further studies, including clarification of the molecular pathways driving EATL pathogenesis, may lead to the development of innovative and more effective treatment modalities for the management of this clinically challengingT-cell lymphoma.

REFERENCES

[1] Ashton-Key, M., et al., Molecular analysis of T-cell clonality in ulcerative jejunitis and enteropathy-associated T-cell lymphoma. *Am. J. Pathol.*, 1997. 151(2): p. 493-8.

[2] Ferreri, A. J., et al., Enteropathy-associated T-cell lymphoma. *Crit. Rev. Oncol. Hematol.*, 2011. 79(1): p. 84-90.

[3] Delabie, J., et al., Enteropathy-associated T-cell lymphoma: clinical and histological findings from the international peripheral T-cell lymphoma project. *Blood*, 2011. 118(1): p. 148-55.

[4] Shack, L. G., et al., Small intestinal cancer in England and Wales and Scotland: time trends in incidence, mortality and survival. *Aliment Pharmacol. Ther.*, 2006. 23(9): p. 1297-306.

[5] Verbeek, W. H., et al., Incidence of enteropathy--associated T-cell lymphoma: a nation-wide study of a population-based registry in The Netherlands. *Scand. J. Gastroenterol.*, 2008. 43(11): p. 1322-8.

[6] Sharaiha, R. Z., et al., Increasing incidence of enteropathy-associated T-cell lymphoma in the United States, 1973-2008. *Cancer*, 2011.

[7] O'Farrelly, C., et al., Humoral response to wheat protein in patients with coeliac disease and enteropathy associated T cell lymphoma. *Br. Med. J.* (Clin. Res. Ed.), 1986. 293(6552): p. 908-10.

[8] Isaacson, P. and D. H. Wright, Intestinal lymphoma associated with malabsorption. *Lancet*, 1978. 1(8055): p. 67-70.

[9] Gough, K. R., A. E. Read, and J. M. Naish, Intestinal reticulosis as a complication of idiopathic steatorrhoea. *Gut*. 1962. 3: p. 232-9.

[10] Deleeuw, R. J., et al., Whole-genome analysis and H. L. A. genotyping of enteropathy-type T-cell lymphoma reveals 2 distinct lymphoma subtypes. *Gastroenterology*, 2007. 132(5): p. 1902-11.

[11] Ko, Y. H., et al., Enteropathy-associated T-cell lymphoma--a clinicopathologic and array comparative genomic hybridization study. *Hum. Pathol.*, 2010. 41(9): p. 1231-7.

[12] Zettl, A., et al., Enteropathy-type T-cell lymphoma. *Am. J. Clin. Pathol.*, 2007. 127(5): p. 701-6.

[13] Baumgartner, A. K., et al., High frequency of genetic aberrations in enteropathy-type T-cell lymphoma. Laboratory investigation; *a journal of technical methods and pathology*, 2003. 83(10): p. 1509-16.

[14] Akiyama, T., et al., CD8+, CD56+ (natural killer-like) T-cell lymphoma involving the small intestine with no evidence of enteropathy: clinicopathology and molecular study of five Japanese patients. *Pathol. Int.*, 2008. 58(10): p. 626-34.

[15] Chuang, S. S. and Y. C. Jung, Natural killer cell lymphoma of small intestine with features of enteropathy but lack of association with celiac disease. *Hum Pathol.*, 2004. 35(5): p. 639-42.

[16] Swerdlow, S. H., International Agency for Research on Cancer., and World Health Organization., *W. H. O. classification of tumours of haematopoietic and lymphoid tissues.* 4th ed. World Health Organization classification of tumours. 2008, Lyon, France: International Agency for Research on Cancer. 439 p.

[17] Di Sabatino, A., et al., How I treat enteropathy-associated T-cell lymphoma. *Blood*, 2012. 119(11): p. 2458-68.

[18] Tack, G. J., et al., Origin and immunophenotype of aberrant I. E. L. in RCDII patients. *Mol. Immunol.*, 2012. 50(4): p. 262-70.

[19] Verkarre, V., et al., Refractory coeliac sprue is a diffuse gastrointestinal disease. *Gut.*, 2003. 52(2): p. 205-11.

[20] Domizio, P., et al., Primary lymphoma of the small intestine. A clinicopathological study of 119 cases. *Am. J. Surg. Pathol.*, 1993. 17(5): p. 429-42.

[21] Chott, A., et al., Classification of intestinal T-cell neoplasms and their differential diagnosis. *Am. J. Clin. Pathol.*, 1999. 111(1 Suppl. 1): p. S68-74.

[22] Bagdi, E., et al., Mucosal intra-epithelial lymphocytes in enteropathy-associated T-cell lymphoma, ulcerative jejunitis, and refractory celiac disease constitute a neoplastic population. *Blood*, 1999. 94(1): p. 260-4.

[23] Chott, A., et al., Most CD56+ intestinal lymphomas are CD8+CD5-T-cell lymphomas of monomorphic small to medium size histology. *Am. J. Pathol.*, 1998. 153(5): p. 1483-90.

[24] Takeshita, M., et al., Pathological and immunohistological findings and genetic aberrations of intestinal enteropathy-associated T cell lymphoma in Japan. *Histopathology,* 2011. 58(3): p. 395-407.

[25] Sun, J., et al., Primary intestinal T-cell and NK-cell lymphomas: a clinicopathological and molecular study from China focused on type II enteropathy-associated T-cell lymphoma and primary intestinal NK-cell lymphoma. *Mod. Pathol.*, 2011. 24(7): p. 983-92.

[26] Ghodke, Y., et al., H. L. A. and disease. *Eur. J. Epidemiol.*, 2005. 20(6): p. 475-88.

[27] Howell, W. M., et al., HLA-DRB, -DQA, and -DQB polymorphism in celiac disease and enteropathy-associated T-cell lymphoma. Common features and additional risk factors for malignancy. *Hum. Immunol.*, 1995. 43(1): p. 29-37.

[28] Kohonen-Corish, M. R., H. Dunckley, and S. W. Serjeantson, HLA-DR and -DQ DNA genotyping in seven populations of Asia-Oceania and Australia. *Tissue Antigens*, 1988. 32(1): p. 32-40.

[29] Chan, J. K., et al., Type II enteropathy-associated T-cell lymphoma: a distinct aggressive lymphoma with frequent gamma delta T-cell receptor expression. *Am. J. Surg. Pathol.*, 2011. 35(10): p. 1557-69.

[30] Lee, K. W., et al., Allelic and haplotypic diversity of HLA-A, -B, -C, -DRB1, and -DQB1 genes in the Korean population. *Tissue Antigens*, 2005. 65(5): p. 437-47.

[31] Saito, S., et al., Allele frequencies and haplotypic associations defined by allelic DNA. typing at H. L. A. class I and class II loci in the Japanese population. *Tissue Antigens*, 2000. 56(6): p. 522-9.

[32] Zettl, A., et al., Chromosomal gains at 9q characterize enteropathy-type T-cell lymphoma. *Am. J. Pathol.*, 2002. 161(5): p. 1635-45.

[33] Sood, A., et al., Increasing incidence of celiac disease in India. *Am. J. Gastroenterol.*, 2001. 96(9): p. 2804-5.

[34] Rubio-Tapia, A., et al., Increased prevalence and mortality in undiagnosed celiac disease. *Gastroenterology*, 2009. 137(1): p. 88-93.

[35] Cataldo, F. and G. Montalto, Celiac disease in the developing countries: a new and challenging public health problem. *World J. Gastroenterol.*, 2007. 13(15): p. 2153-9.

[36] Lohi, S., et al., Increasing prevalence of coeliac disease over time. *Aliment Pharmacol. Ther.*, 2007. 26(9): p. 1217-25.

[37] van den Broeck, H. C., et al., Presence of celiac disease epitopes in modern and old hexaploid wheat varieties: wheat breeding may have contributed to increased prevalence of celiac disease. *Theor. Appl. Genet.*, 2010. 121(8): p. 1527-39.

[38] Altpeter, F., et al., Integration and expression of the high-molecular-weight glutenin subunit 1Ax1 gene into wheat. *Nat. Biotechnol.*, 1996. 14(9): p. 1155-9.

[39] Blechl, A. E. and O. D. Anderson, Expression of a novel high-molecular-weight glutenin subunit gene in transgenic wheat. *Nat. Biotechnol.*, 1996. 14(7): p. 875-9.

[40] Field, J. M., et al., Introgression of transgenes into a commercial cultivar confirms differential effects of HMW subunits 1Ax1 and 1Dx5 on gluten properties. *Journal of Cereal Science*, 2008. 48(2): p. 457-463.

[41] Agriculture, US. Do. Wheat's Role in the US Diet Has Changed Over the Decades 2009; Available from: *http://www.ers.usda.gov/briefing/wheat/consumption.htm.*

[42] Green, P. H. and C. Cellier, Celiac disease. *N. Engl. J. Med.*, 2007. 357(17): p. 1731-43.

[43] Malamut, G., et al., IL-15 triggers an antiapoptotic pathway in human intraepithelial lymphocytes that is a potential new target in celiac disease-associated inflammation and lymphomagenesis. *J. Clin. Invest.*, 2010. 120(6): p. 2131-43.

[44] Rubio-Tapia, A. and J. A. Murray, Classification and management of refractory coeliac disease. *Gut.*, 2010. 59(4): p. 547-57.

[45] Tack, G. J., et al., The spectrum of celiac disease: epidemiology, clinical aspects and treatment. *Nat. Rev. Gastroenterol. Hepatol.*, 2010. 7(4): p. 204-13.

[46] Biagi, F. and G. R. Corazza, Mortality in celiac disease. *Nat. Rev. Gastroenterol. Hepatol.*, 2010. 7(3): p. 158-62.

[47] Van Belzen, M. J., et al., A major non-HLA locus in celiac disease maps to chromosome 19. *Gastroenterology*, 2003. 125(4): p. 1032-41.

[48] Wolters, V. M. and C. Wijmenga, Genetic background of celiac disease and its clinical implications. *Am. J. Gastroenterol.*, 2008. 103(1): p. 190-5.

[49] Woolley, N., et al., A new locus for coeliac disease mapped to chromosome 15 in a population isolate. *Hum. Genet.*, 2002. 111(1): p. 40-5.

[50] Greco, L., et al., Existence of a genetic risk factor on chromosome 5q in Italian coeliac disease families. *Ann. Hum. Genet.,* 2001. 65(Pt 1): p. 35-41.

[51] Jiang, W., et al., c-Myc controls the development of CD8alphaalpha TCRalphabeta intestinal intraepithelial lymphocytes from thymic precursors by regulating IL-15-dependent survival. *Blood,* 2010. 115(22): p. 4431-8.

[52] Gale, J., et al., Enteropathy-type intestinal T-cell lymphoma: clinical features and treatment of 31 patients in a single center. *J. Clin. Oncol.*, 2000. 18(4): p. 795-803.

[53] Novakovic, B. J., S. Novakovic, and S. Frkovic-Grazio, A single-center report on clinical features and treatment response in patients with intestinal T cell non-Hodgkin's lymphomas. *Oncol. Rep.*, 2006. 16(1): p. 191-5.

[54] Sieniawski, M. K. and A. L. Lennard, Enteropathy-associated T-cell lymphoma: epidemiology, clinical features, and current treatment strategies. *Curr. Hematol. Malig. Rep.*, 2011. 6(4): p. 231-40.

[55] Daum, S., et al., Intestinal non-Hodgkin's lymphoma: a multicenter prospective clinical study from the German Study Group on Intestinal non-Hodgkin's Lymphoma. *J. Clin. Oncol.*, 2003. 21(14): p. 2740-6.

[56] Tse, E., et al., Type II enteropathy associated t-cell lymphoma: A multi center analysis from the Asia Lymphoma Study Group. *American Journal of Hematology*, 2012: p. n/a-n/a.

[57] Deguchi, Y., K. Yoshimatsu, and S. Endo, Natural killer-like T cell lymphoma of the small intestine: report of a case. *Surg. Today*, 2006. 36(5): p. 474-7.

[58] N C C N. Guidelines Non Hodgkin Lymphoma Version 2.2012. 2012.

[59] Laird, J., M. Leach, and S. Ballantyne, The value of small bowel magnetic resonance imaging in the management of enteropathy associated T-cell lymphoma. *Br. J. Haematol.*, 2008. 142(1): p. 136-7.

[60] Van Weyenberg, S. J., et al., M. R. enteroclysis in refractory celiac disease: proposal and validation of a severity scoring system. *Radiology*, 2011. 259(1): p. 151-61.

[61] Fry, L. C., et al., Utility of double-balloon enteroscopy for the evaluation of malabsorption. *Dig. Dis.*, 2008. 26(2): p. 134-9.

[62] Beaton, C., M. Davies, and J. Beynon, The management of primary small bowel and colon lymphoma-a review. *Int. J. Colorectal. Dis.*, 2011.

[63] Kakugawa, Y., et al., Enteropathy-associated T-cell lymphoma in small intestine detected by capsule endoscopy. *Leuk. Lymphoma*, 2012.

[64] Goetz, M. and T. D. Wang, Molecular imaging in gastrointestinal endoscopy. *Gastroenterology*, 2010. 138(3): p. 828-33 e1.

[65] Goetz, M. and R. Kiesslich, Advances of endomicroscopy for gastrointestinal physiology and diseases. *Am. J. Physiol. Gastrointest. Liver Physiol.*, 2010. 298(6): p. G797-806.

[66] Rohatiner, A., et al., Report on a workshop convened to discuss the pathological and staging classifications of gastrointestinal tract lymphoma. *Ann. Oncol.*, 1994. 5(5): p. 397-400.

[67] A predictive model for aggressive non-Hodgkin's lymphoma. The International Non-Hodgkin's Lymphoma Prognostic Factors Project. *N. Engl. J. Med.*, 1993. 329(14): p. 987-94.

[68] Gallamini, A., et al., Peripheral T-cell lymphoma unspecified (PTCL-U): a new prognostic model from a retrospective multicentric clinical study. *Blood*, 2004. 103(7): p. 2474-9.

[69] Wada, M., et al., Spontaneous gastrointestinal perforation in patients with lymphoma receiving chemotherapy and steroids. Report of three cases. *Nihon Ika Daigaku Zasshi*, 1999. 66(1): p. 37-40.

[70] Egan, L. J., et al., Celiac-associated lymphoma. A single institution experience of 30 cases in the combination chemotherapy era. *J. Clin. Gastroenterol.*, 1995. 21(2): p. 123-9.

[71] Raderer, M., et al., Second line chemotherapy in patients with enteropathy-associated T cell lymphoma: a retrospective single center analysis. *Ann. Hematol.*, 2012. 91(1): p. 57-61.

[72] Honemann, D., et al., Enteropathy-associated T-cell lymphoma without a prior diagnosis of coeliac disease: diagnostic dilemmas and management options. *Ann. Hematol.*, 2005. 84(2): p. 118-21.

[73] Morton, J. E., et al., Primary gastrointestinal non-Hodgkin's lymphoma: a review of 175 British National Lymphoma Investigation cases. *Br. J. Cancer*, 1993. 67(4): p. 776-82.

[74] Wohrer, S., et al., Chemotherapy with cyclophosphamide, doxorubicin, etoposide, vincristine and prednisone (C. H. O. E. P.) is not effective in patients with enteropathy-type intestinal T-cell lymphoma. *Ann. Oncol.*, 2004. 15(11): p. 1680-3.

[75] Sieniawski, M., et al., Evaluation of enteropathy-associated T-cell lymphoma comparing standard therapies with a novel regimen including autologous stem cell transplantation. *Blood*, 2010. 115(18): p. 3664-70.

[76] Al-Toma, A. and C. J. Mulder, Review article: Stem cell transplantation for the treatment of gastrointestinal diseases--current applications and future perspectives. *Aliment Pharmacol. Ther.*, 2007. 26 Suppl. 2: p. 77-89.

[77] Jantunen, E., et al., High-dose therapy supported by autologous stem cell transplantation in patients with enteropathy-associated T-cell lymphoma. *Leuk. Lymphoma*, 2003. 44(12): p. 2163-4.

[78] Bishton, M. J. and A. P. Haynes, Combination chemotherapy followed by autologous stem cell transplant for enteropathy-associated T cell lymphoma. *Br. J. Haematol.*, 2007. 136(1): p. 111-3.

[79] Al-Toma, A., et al., Disappointing outcome of autologous stem cell transplantation for enteropathy-associated T-cell lymphoma. *Dig. Liver Dis.*, 2007. 39(7): p. 634-41.

[80] Reimer, P., et al., Autologous stem-cell transplantation as first-line therapy in peripheral T-cell lymphomas: results of a prospective multicenter study. *J. Clin. Oncol.*, 2009. 27(1): p. 106-13.

[81] Rongey, C., et al., Successful treatment of enteropathy-associated T cell lymphoma with autologous stem cell transplant. *Dig. Dis. Sci.*, 2006. 51(6): p. 1082-6.

[82] Blystad, A. K., et al., High-dose therapy with autologous stem cell transplantation in patients with peripheral T cell lymphomas. *Bone Marrow Transplant*, 2001. 27(7): p. 711-6.

[83] Gallamini, A., et al., Alemtuzumab (Campath-1H) and CHOP. chemotherapy as first-line treatment of peripheral T-cell lymphoma: results of a G. I. T. I. L. (Gruppo Italiano Terapie Innovative nei Linfomi) prospective multicenter trial. *Blood*, 2007. 110(7): p. 2316-23.

[84] Kircher, S. M., S. Gurbuxani, and S. M. Smith, CH OP. plus alemtuzumab can induce metabolic response by F. D. G. - P. E. T. but has minimal long-term benefits: a case report and literature review. *J. Gastrointest. Cancer*, 2007. 38(1): p. 59-62.

[85] Soldini, D., et al., Efficacy of alemtuzumab and gemcitabine in a patient with enteropathy-type T-cell lymphoma. *Br. J. Haematol.*, 2008. 142(3): p. 484-6.

[86] Piekarz, R. L., et al., Phase 2 trial of romidepsin in patients with peripheral T-cell lymphoma. *Blood*, 2011. 117(22): p. 5827-34.

INDEX

#

A

B

C

D

E

F

G

H

I

N

O

P

Q

R

S

T

U

V

W

Y